THE HEALTHY BARIATRIC SMOOTHIES RECIPE BOOK

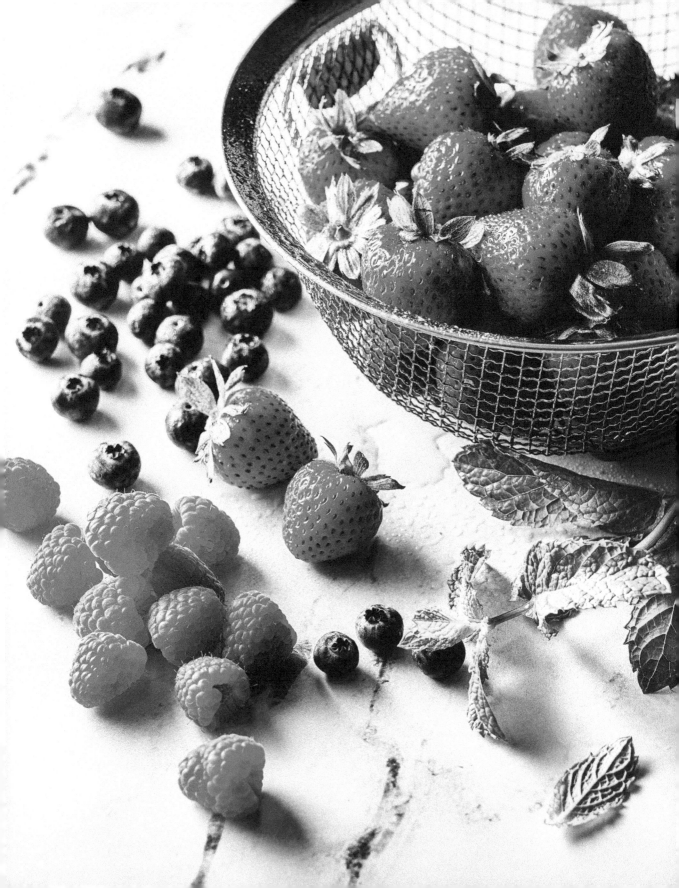

THE HEALTHY BARIATRIC SMOOTHIES RECIPE BOOK

60 NOURISHING HIGH-PROTEIN SMOOTHIES AND SHAKES

STACI GULBIN, MS, MEd, RD

ROCKRIDGE
PRESS

Interior and Cover Designer: Irene Vandervoort
Art Producer: Samantha Ulban
Editor: Anne Goldberg
Production Editor: Ruth Sakata Corley
Production Manager: Eric Pier-Hocking

Photography © Pixle Stories/Stocksy, Cover; Thomas J. Story, p.ii; Evi Abeler, pp. viii, 36; Annie Martin, p.18; StockFood / für ZS Verlag / Kramp + Gölling, p.54; StockFood / Timmann, Claudia, p.72; Hélène Dujardin, p.90

Author photo courtesy of D Taylor Images

Paperback ISBN: 978-1-63878-707-5
eBook ISBN: 978-1-63878-542-2
R0

Contents

Introduction

Welcome to *The Healthy Bariatric Smoothies Recipe Book*!

My name is Staci Gulbin, and I've been a registered dietitian for over 10 years. As a bariatric dietitian, counselor, and health educator, I worked with patients who were in the process of deciding whether they wanted to undergo bariatric surgery, those who were meeting with me to prepare for surgery, and patients who were in the post-op stages of surgery recovery.

Bariatric surgery is a major procedure that requires life changes in what you eat, when you eat, and how you eat while also ensuring that you take in enough daily nutrients for optimal recovery and overall health. Getting enough nutrition each day is vital to avoiding post-op health issues like hair loss and nutrient deficiencies and bone health issues like osteoporosis.

Before surgery, it's important to find flavors and textures that you enjoy so you will know how to plan meals after surgery. It will also be important to learn ways to consume enough protein in small portions and to have a plan in place to ensure that you eat enough protein daily as that will be a top priority after surgery.

In the early stages after surgery, it can be difficult to meet your dietary needs since your digestive system will work a bit differently than it did before. You will need to consume smoother textures for the first several months to help your altered system get used to digesting foods again. You will only be able to tolerate small portions of food at a time, so you will need to eat more slowly and space meals out throughout the day.

Smoothies are a great tool to help ensure that you get adequate daily nutrients. They also provide an easy-to-digest meal that is safe for any stage after bariatric surgery (with the exception of the clear liquid phase, of course). The combinations of flavors are nearly endless, as are the protein sources you can use to create flavorful, smooth drinks to please your taste buds while helping you meet your daily nutrient needs.

This cookbook will save you from having to search on the internet for the perfect smoothie recipe or blindly blend combinations of ingredients on your own. The 60 smoothie recipes in this book have been specially formulated to provide bariatric patients with the appropriate nutrients to meet their nutritional needs while providing an array of flavor profiles to keep meals from becoming boring.

Each smoothie uses minimally processed foods along with herbs, spices, and protein-rich bases to create ideal meal replacements and healthy snacks. And to ensure that the smoothie recipes fit within your pre-op and post-op meal plans, they are low in calories and high in hydration and contain low amounts of added sugar.

No matter what stage pre-surgery or post-surgery you are in, this cookbook is designed to be a great resource to provide the basics regarding your nutrient needs. It provides step-by-step instructions on how to prepare your kitchen so your pantry and refrigerator will contain all the ingredients you need to create delicious and nutritious smoothies any time of day.

A bariatric surgery journey may not be an easy one, but it is one in which you will be taking brave steps to change your health for the better. Congratulations to you and the best of luck as you become the healthier you that you deserve to be. May this book help you make that journey a smooth, successful, and flavorful one.

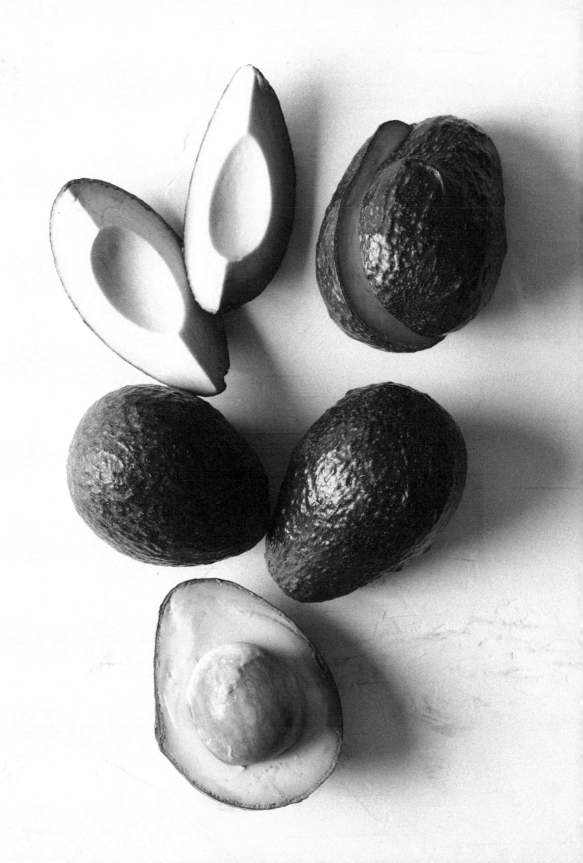

1

YOUR SMOOTHIE KITCHEN

The bariatric diet is a challenging eating plan, not only because you have to limit sugar and fat but also because of the texture stages you must follow post-op. At times during the first three to six months, you may start to crave more solid foods, which can make complying with the meal plan difficult. You may think you have to live on prepackaged protein drinks and sugar-free puddings for months. But including a variety of flavorful smoothies in your meal plan will help you survive the early stages of the journey.

This chapter will teach you all you need to know about which textures you can eat in the early stages after surgery, the nutrients you need each day, and how to prepare your kitchen for making the most delicious smoothies, morning, noon, or night.

DIET AND YOUR BARIATRIC JOURNEY

For the first three to six months after bariatric surgery, you will have to consume soft food textures, starting with clear liquids and gradually moving to full liquids before eating puréed textures. Usually, solid foods won't come into the picture until closer to six months after surgery.

At each stage you will also have a different set of calories and nutrients that you must eat to ensure that your body obtains what it needs to heal from surgery and to experience a successful health outcome. Continue reading to learn more about the guidelines for pre-op as well as the various texture stages of the post-op bariatric diet.

PRE-OP

There are no specific texture restrictions before surgery, but your surgeon will likely place you on a diet for at least two weeks ahead to help shrink your liver. This will provide your surgeon greater access to your stomach and intestines and ensure a safer outcome. During the pre-op diet, you will consume mostly protein shakes, along with one or two small low-carbohydrate and high-protein meals.

POST-OP

Depending on the type of surgery you receive, your post-op diet schedule may differ slightly from what I relay here. However, all patients will start with clear liquids like broths, herbal teas, and clear protein drinks. They will slowly move up to full liquids like milk, plant-based milk, and protein shakes as well as cream-based broths, for example. After tolerating full liquids, the patient will consume puréed textures such as blended fruits and vegetables, including mashed potatoes, smoothies, puddings, and yogurt. Once the puréed texture is tolerated, the patient will slowly graduate to solid foods.

GASTRIC BYPASS

Weeks 1 and 2: Clear liquids

Weeks 3 and 4: Purées (introduce protein supplements)

Months 2 and 3: Soft foods

Months 4 and beyond: Stabilization/general diet

ADJUSTABLE GASTRIC BAND

Week 1: Clear liquids

Week 2: All liquids (introduce protein supplements)

Week 3: Purées

Weeks 4 and 5: Soft foods

Week 6 and beyond: Stabilization/general diet

BARIATRIC NUTRITIONAL KNOW-HOW

After surgery, you will need to follow certain nutritional guidelines to ensure that your body receives what it needs for healing. You will also need to limit some nutrients like sugar and fat that may trigger negative symptoms with your newly altered digestive system, including nausea, vomiting, diarrhea, and abdominal pain. Each nutrient has specific functions and guidelines in your post-operative diet.

PROTEIN

Protein is a vital nutrient to consume before but especially after surgery to help preserve lean muscle mass and assist with healing. During each post-op stage, you will slowly increase your daily protein intake as you are able to tolerate a bit more volume at each meal.

LIQUID PHASE: 50 to 70 grams daily

PURÉED FOODS: 50 to 70 grams daily

SOFT FOODS: 60 to 80 grams daily

GENERAL FOODS: 60 to 100 grams daily

Research shows that those who have had bariatric surgery should follow a high-protein diet with foods that contain about 35 percent of calories from protein. For a 1,000-calorie diet, which is typical of the early stages post-op, you will consume foods containing a total of about 350 calories from protein. Since each gram of protein contains about 4 calories, this comes out to about 87.5 grams of protein, which is within the range of what is recommended for optimal health post-op.

FAT

The post-op guidelines for fat intake apply universally throughout the texture stages. Those who have had sleeve gastrectomy or Roux-en-Y surgery should consume no more than 20 percent of their calories from fat. Therefore, if you follow a 1,000-calorie diet, you should consume no more than 200 calories from fat each day. One gram of fat is equal to 9 calories. For this calorie amount, you should stick to about 22 grams of fat daily.

This lower fat intake will not only help prevent weight gain over the long term it will also reduce the risk for fat intolerance symptoms such as abdominal pain, diarrhea, and nausea. To stay within this limit, try to stick to no more than 5 grams of fat per serving per meal.

CARBOHYDRATE

Research shows that those who have had sleeve gastrectomy or Roux-en-Y surgery should consume between 35 percent and 48 percent of their calories from carbohydrates daily.

After bariatric surgery, you will have to follow a fairly low-carbohydrate diet that does not exceed 130 grams of carbohydrates daily. Research shows you should consume about 40 percent of your calories from carbohydrates for optimal, long-term weight loss success. For example, if you consume 1200 calories daily, you should consume no more than 40 percent, or 480 calories, from carbohydrates daily. Each gram of carbohydrate is equal to about 4 calories, so that comes out to about 120 grams of carbohydrates daily.

SUGAR

After bariatric surgery, you should limit sugar as much as possible to reduce the risk of "dumping syndrome," which can cause uncomfortable symptoms such as nausea, vomiting, diarrhea, and abdominal pain. The American Society for Metabolic and Bariatric Surgery recommends that post-op patients consume foods that contain no more than 15 grams of sugar per serving.

Be sure to limit sugar alcohol intake to no more than 10 grams per serving. Sugar alcohols include ingredients such as xylitol, maltitol, and sorbitol. Although they are found in sugar-free products, they can cause uncomfortable digestive symptoms if consumed in excess.

MINERALS AND OTHER NUTRIENTS

Because your overall consumption is limited after surgery, taking supplements of vitamins, minerals, and other nutrients is encouraged to bolster the small quantities available in your diet. For all post-op phases, it is recommended that you consume:

- A multivitamin
- Calcium (at least 1,200 milligrams per day)
- Vitamin D (about 1,000 International Units per day)
- Vitamin B_{12} (500 to 1,000 micrograms per day)

This is not a final list because your doctor may recommend you take other daily supplements if you have or are at greater risk for certain nutrient deficiencies.

KEEP HYDRATED!

After surgery, it will be vital to consume plenty of fluids to help maintain hydration. This may be challenging since your stomach will hold much less than it did before surgery. The guidelines for post-op liquid consumption are 48 to 64 ounces daily during both the clear liquid and full liquid phases and 64 or more ounces, as tolerated, during the puréed, soft food, and general food phases. To avoid digestive discomfort, it's important to follow the guidelines here when planning your fluid intake after bariatric surgery.

- Do not drink fluids within 30 minutes before and 30 minutes after eating.

- Do not consume carbonated drinks or chew gum since both can allow air to enter the pouch of your stomach, which can cause pain and discomfort.

- Avoid using straws after bariatric surgery since they can cause air to enter the pouch. This can lead to abdominal pain and can also take up space in your smaller stomach that you need for your new high-protein diet.

- Drink slowly with small sips of no more than an ounce or two at a time. It can help to have a water bottle that is marked with measurements on the side so you can keep track of how much you are drinking each time you drink as well as your total intake throughout the day.

MAKING SMOOTHIES PART OF YOUR DAILY DIET

Smoothies and shakes are a convenient and easily digestible meal or snack option for those on a pre-op or post-op bariatric diet—aside from during the clear liquid phase, of course. Here are my top five reasons to incorporate smoothies into your bariatric diet:

1. **Smoothies make for quick meal prep.** As long as you have the proper ingredients on hand, you can make a smoothie in less than five minutes. Just chop up some veggies or fruit, throw them in the blender with your preferred protein source, pour in some liquid and maybe some ice, and blend.

2. **Smoothies are convenient and portable.** Once you make your smoothie, you can just pour it into any cup or mug with a lid and take it with you during your busy day. Smoothies can help you stay healthy no matter how hectic your schedule becomes.

3. **Your body can easily digest smoothies.** Because smoothies are made from blended ingredients, there is not much left for your body to break down. For someone with an altered digestive system, like those who have had bariatric surgery, smoothies give your body a break while still providing needed nutrients.

4. **Smoothies do double duty.** Smoothies can provide antioxidants from leafy greens or brightly colored berries, plus they can give you fiber from fruits, vegetables, nut butters, and seeds. You can also get protein from yogurt, soy milk, or protein powder that are often added to smoothies. In addition to all the nutrients they can provide, smoothies provide an adequate source of hydration to keep your organs functioning properly.

5. **Easy for all skill levels.** No matter what your level of cooking skill, making smoothies requires the most basic of chopping and measuring abilities. If you know how to use a vegetable peeler, rinse off produce, and use measuring cups and spoons, then you can make a smoothie.

SMOOTHIE CENTRAL

In order to make delicious and nutritious smoothies anytime you want, you need to make sure your kitchen is always at the ready. Not only do you need a blender, you should also make sure you have all the smoothie staples on hand to make a drink that is balanced in both flavor and nutrition.

THE BLENDER

You could have all the fresh produce in the world, but if you don't have a blender, it will be nearly impossible to create a properly smooth smoothie. There's no need to spend hundreds of dollars, but whatever you choose, it should have certain characteristics that will be able to stand up to a daily smoothie-making routine.

MULTIPLE SPEEDS

Be sure that the blender you choose has a variety of blending speeds so you can customize based on what type of smoothie you want to make. Some portable blenders may seem convenient since you can make and drink your smoothie in the same cup, but if they only offer one speed, they will likely not be powerful enough to crush ice or seeds or create a smooth enough texture to accommodate your post-op bariatric diet needs. Choose a blender that has at least three speeds.

ICE-CRUSHING POWER

Read reviews and, if possible, ask for a demonstration of the blender you are thinking of buying to make sure it crushes ice well. The blender you choose should have sharp blades to grind ice into a snow-like texture so your smoothies can provide adequate thickness and consistency.

EASY TO CLEAN

Since you will be using your blender pretty much every day after surgery, it's important to have one that is easy to clean. This means your blender should have an easily removable and replaceable blade, an easy-to-clean base, and a container that is either dishwasher safe or easy to clean by hand.

DURABILITY

For daily use, you will need a model that is durable. You may want to choose a blender with a container that is made of thick and durable plastic rather than heavy or bulky glass containers that might easily crack or break.

THE INGREDIENTS

To concoct a smoothie that is balanced in both flavor and nutrition, you must include a source of fiber, a liquid, a flavoring, and a source of protein. It's good to keep a variety of ingredients on hand to make sure you always have what you need from each category. Right after surgery, although protein is a priority, hydration and fiber are also important to optimal health. Therefore, chapter 2 will include smoothies with a more fluid base. Take note that these smoothies will have less protein.

PROTEIN POWDER

You can add protein powder to almost any of the smoothies if you are looking for a way to increase protein in an easy-to-digest form. This is especially helpful during the first three months or so after bariatric surgery when you cannot tolerate solid foods. It's also great for a quick portable protein source before or after a workout.

When choosing a protein powder, try to select one with the fewest ingredients. For example, buy a whey protein powder made from 100 percent whey protein or a plant-based protein powder containing just pea or rice proteins. When choosing a protein powder, avoid any with added sugars, artificial flavors, and artificial sweeteners.

You should be aware that although common ingredients in protein powders such as sunflower lecithin and gums may sound unnatural, they are safe to consume. These ingredients are simply plant-based compounds that help the proteins and fats in a protein powder bind together well so your drink will have a smooth and creamy texture. Some people may experience gastrointestinal distress after consuming certain gums, but overall, they are safe to consume, and a 2019 study in the journal *Nutrients* shows they may even help reduce blood glucose levels.

My favorite brand of protein powder that meets such guidelines is TGS 100% Whey Protein Powder. It's great for when you want to add protein to a smoothie without adding any additional flavor.

DAIRY

If you're not keen on using protein powder in your smoothie but you still want to add a bit of protein to your drink, try adding milk or yogurt. Be sure to use unsweetened dairy products so you can better control the sugar content of your smoothie. And when it comes to yogurt, use Greek yogurt for the most protein-dense option.

NONDAIRY

If you prefer a nondairy smoothie, use plant-based milks like unsweetened almond, coconut, or cashew milk. For a little extra protein, try soy milk. Plant-based yogurts are an option for adding creaminess, but since they tend to contain less protein, try blending in some soft tofu to your smoothie for a smooth texture.

FRUIT

When choosing fruit for your smoothie, there are many options. What you select will depend on what flavor profile you are looking for, but in general, you should seek out fruits with lower carbohydrates, such as these:

- Avocados
- Berries (blueberries, strawberries, blackberries, or raspberries)
- Kiwi
- Melons (watermelon, cantaloupe, or honeydew)
- Peaches

If you prefer to have fruit on hand to have smoothies anytime but are not sure if you will be able to consume it all before it spoils, buy frozen, unsweetened fruit, which will work just fine. Canned fruit is also good to use as long as it contains no added sugar.

VEGETABLES, LEAFY GREENS, AND FRESH HERBS

For added fiber and antioxidants, fresh herbs and vegetables are great additions, including these:

- Baby spinach leaves
- Basil
- Beets
- Carrots
- Cilantro
- Cucumbers (peeled and seeded to reduce bitterness)
- Mint leaves

Although vegetables are good for you, your body will not tolerate raw fruits and vegetables very well during the first three months after surgery, so if you use them, be sure to blend them extremely well until completely smooth and then strain out any remaining solid fibrous pieces.

To strain blended vegetables: Place a fine-mesh strainer over a small to medium bowl. Pour the blended smoothie into the strainer and, using the back of a spoon, press the mixture through the strainer until as much of the liquid is squeezed out as possible. This will take about three minutes. Discard any seeds or other solids, pour the liquid into a glass, and enjoy.

FLAVORINGS

To add even more flavor to your smoothies, try mixing in some alcohol-free vanilla or almond extract, or add some cocoa powder for a rich chocolate flavor. Adding unsweetened coconut milk will also add a bit of natural coconut flavor. Ground spices like cinnamon, ginger, and turmeric can add antioxidants as well as great flavor.

OTHER INGREDIENTS

Other ingredients that can provide depth of flavor as well as an extra kick of nutrition include these:

- Citrus juices (lemons, limes, oranges, clementines, or grapefruits)

- Green tea (extra antioxidants, flavor, and caffeine)

- Ground flaxseed (extra protein, fiber, and omega-3 fatty acids)

- Ice (extra hydration)

- Natural sweeteners (stevia, pure maple syrup, or honey)

- Nut butters (peanut butter or almond butter)

- Oats (extra fiber and a thickener)

INGREDIENTS TO AVOID

If you're trying to lower your carbohydrate intake, limit the addition of the following higher-sugar ingredients to your smoothies or choose recipes without them.

- **Dates:** One date contains 16 grams of sugar.

- **Fruit juices like apple or grape juice:** One cup of apple juice contains 24 grams of sugar, and one cup of grape juice contains 36 grams of sugar.

LEARNING TO LOVE
NATURAL SWEETNESS

I t's important to reduce your sugar intake after bariatric surgery. This is because in some people, especially those who have had Roux-en-Y surgery, higher sugar intakes can lead to a condition known as "dumping syndrome" in which large amounts of food, especially sugar, move quickly from the stomach to the small intestine, causing abdominal cramping, diarrhea, nausea, or vomiting.

One thing you can do prior to surgery to lower the risk of dumping syndrome is to try to reduce your cravings by cutting out foods that are high in sugar. This includes some fruits and other natural sources of sugars such as dairy products. Research, including a study published in *The Permanente Journal*, shows that after about a week of avoiding sugary foods and drinks (including those with artificial sweeteners), many people stop craving sweets.

You'll find that most of the flavor in the smoothie recipes in this book comes from low-carbohydrate fruits and vegetables as well as from a natural sweetener known as stevia extract. Studies show that stevia extract does not increase blood glucose levels after eating and does not further increase food intake, making it a great natural alternative to sugar to help sweeten your foods and drinks without increasing your craving for sugar. My favorite brand of stevia is Splenda Stevia Naturals.

SMOOTHIE MAKING 101

When making a smoothie, it's important to decide first what texture you desire, which will help you determine what ingredients to use. If you prefer a thinner smoothie that you can easily pour, use a liquid base such as milk or water. If you prefer a smoothie that's thick enough to stand your spoon in, then use yogurt and some ice instead. If you prefer, you could use frozen fruit instead of ice for this thicker smoothie texture.

You should also be aware that the order of ingredients placed in the blender matters when it comes to smoothie consistency.

1. First, pour the liquid (milk, water) or semisolid (yogurt, cottage cheese) ingredients into the blender as the base.

2. Add the fruits and/or vegetables as well as any nuts, nut butters, or seeds.

3. Last, add the ice, which will help pull all the other ingredients down into the blades to create an even, and eventually smooth, mixture.

When it comes to which blender speed to use, it will depend on what ingredients you are using in your smoothie. For a smoothie containing extra-fibrous vegetables and fruits as well as those with lots of ice, you may need to use a high speed. For smoothies containing fibrous produce along with a liquid base, a medium speed may be enough to create the smooth, even texture you want. For smoothies containing low-fiber produce, such as berries or peeled cucumber, along with a liquid base, a low speed may be enough.

The blending time may vary depending on the ingredients in your smoothie and the strength of your blender. On average, the recipes in this book will take about 60 seconds of steady blending time to achieve smooth results. Depending on the blender you use, it may take longer to obtain the consistency you are looking for. It's important to watch the blender carefully to ensure that all the ingredients are evenly blended.

To avoid grittiness in your smoothie, mix the protein powder and the liquid or semisolid base in a separate container first before adding it to the blender. You can also use milk or plant-based milk instead of water to get a creamier texture or blend in a creamy fruit like avocado to help smooth out the consistency.

SMOOTHIES (ALMOST) READY WHEN YOU WANT THEM

I f you want to enjoy smoothies often but you don't have the time to prep every day, smoothie freezer packs may become your new best friend. To make them, prep the fruit and vegetables you want to use in your smoothies along with any additional solid ingredients like nuts or spices, and combine them in single-serving zip-top plastic freezer bags before storing in the freezer.

When you are ready to make a smoothie, pour the liquid base ingredients into the blender, add the frozen prepped ingredients, and blend. Because the fruits and/or vegetables are frozen, you probably won't need to put in additional ice, but you can add more ice if desired to get the texture you want. When prepping and freezing, be sure to label the freezer bags so you can decide the best liquid or semisolid base to add.

ABOUT THE RECIPES

The smoothies in this book are ideal for people who are preparing for or have had bariatric surgery, so they all conform to lower-calorie parameters and are low in sugar, nutrient rich, and high in protein. They all contain less than 15 grams of net carbohydrates per serving. (Net carbohydrates are the total grams of carbohydrates minus the grams of fiber because fiber is not technically digested in the body.) The recipes are organized into four chapters, which will make it easy to choose which recipe to make.

REFRESHING

These smoothies provide exactly what the name of this chapter describes: a light and refreshing drink that will help provide hydration. Keep in mind that these recipes won't always contain adequate protein to act as a meal replacement.

CREAMY

This is the chapter to turn to when you have a craving for a rich and creamy dessert. These smoothies will provide a rich and delicious taste, and they are also a good source of protein. Depending on the fruits and/or vegetables used, they also provide a variety of antioxidants.

FRUITY

If you're craving fruit but cannot yet tolerate solid foods, these fruity smoothies are the perfect choice. They contain the refreshing fruits you love and use a milk or plant-based milk base along with other flavors to provide a nutrient-dense, easy-to-digest beverage.

SAVORY

Try one of these smoothies if you'd like to give your palate a unique and delicious experience. Smooth and savory foods are most often served warm or hot in dishes like soup, but these smoothies show that it's possible to enjoy drinking your vegetables, too. The recipes in this chapter are rich in nutrients and can stand in as meal replacements if needed.

Many of the smoothie recipes include tips on how to adjust them to meet your needs. These tips fall into three categories:

POST-OP TIPS

These tips explain how you can change the recipe to meet your post-op needs. They also might caution you about swapping out ingredients on your own because it could impact the nutritional profile or texture of a smoothie in a way that might make the beverage no longer compatible with your post-op needs.

PREP TIPS

Look here for ways to make prepping easier so that smoothie making can become more convenient, which will help you fit smoothies into your life and encourage you to make them more often.

VARIATION TIPS

Here you'll find information on adding or changing ingredients to alter the flavor profile, which could provide more variety to your smoothie routine.

Each smoothie recipe includes nutritional information that tells you the amounts of calories, fat, protein, total carbohydrates, total fiber, sugar, and sodium that each serving contains. You will be able to plan your week with smoothies that meet the nutrient needs you require each day. Each smoothie will have a serving size of about one cup, give or take, a good small amount to ensure it is not too much volume for your body to tolerate after surgery.

All you need to do now is turn the page and enjoy the process of creating and drinking nutritious smoothies that will make your post-op bariatric surgery journey much easier and certainly more delicious.

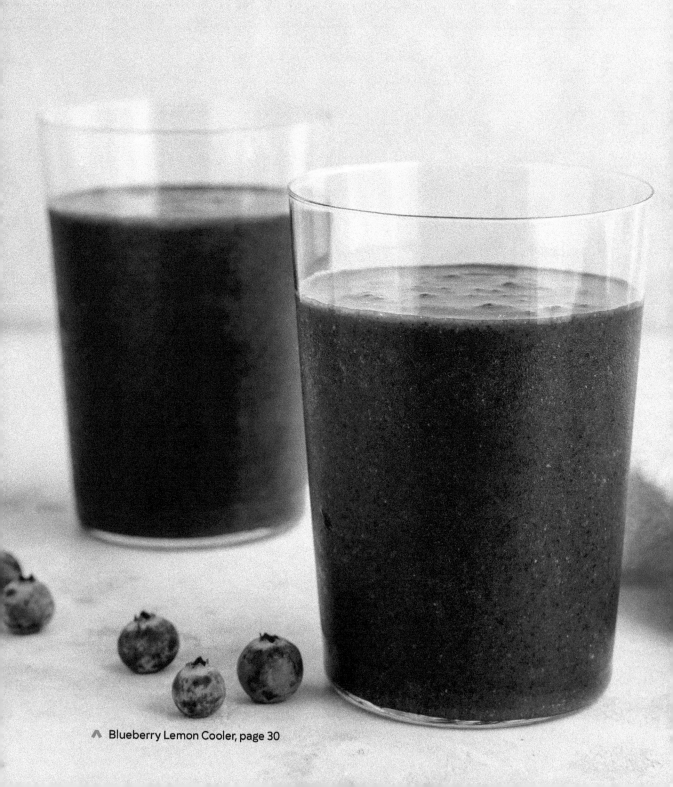

Blueberry Lemon Cooler, page 30

2

REFRESHING

Made with mostly fruit and ice, all these smoothies are ideal at any stage post-op, but they are especially important for immediately after the operation when it's very important to stay hydrated. But honestly, they are great whenever you want a drink that is cooling and thirst-quenching. The recipes in this chapter are not very high in protein, but they can be adapted by using your favorite protein-rich milk, plant-based milk, or protein powder, which will create a more filling smoothie experience. Please note that if you add any of those ingredients to the recipes in this chapter, it will affect the flavor and nutritional content of the final smoothie.

CUCUMBER MINT COOLER

For the ultimate in hydration, this herbal smoothie will soothe your gut with the invigorating flavor of fresh mint and the juiciness of cucumber. Be sure to both peel and remove the seeds from the cucumber before blending because they will be hard to digest post-op and will add a bitter taste to your smoothie.

½ cup cold water

1 cup peeled, seeded, and roughly chopped cucumber

About 6 (1-inch) fresh mint leaves

1 teaspoon stevia or your preferred low-calorie sweetener

1 cup ice

1. In a blender, combine the water, cucumber, mint leaves, stevia, and ice and purée on medium speed until smooth, 60 to 90 seconds.

2. Pour into 2 glasses and enjoy.

3. Store any leftover smoothie in a sealed container, such as a mason jar with a lid, in the refrigerator for up to 2 days. The liquid and solid ingredients will separate and impact the taste and texture, so reblend the smoothie for 10 to 15 seconds before serving.

Per Serving: Calories: 7.5; Fat: 0.1g; Protein: 0.39g; Carbs: 1.9g; Fiber: 0.45g; Sugar: 0.92g; Sodium: 1.33mg

CUCUMBER LIME COOLER

Prep time: 5 minutes   **Yield:** 2 (1-cup) servings

The flavor of lime goes really well with cucumber, making this a really satisfying quencher for pre- or post-op. Anytime you need a zingy pick-me-up or you want to cleanse your palate after a meal, you'll appreciate its refreshing smoothness.

½ cup water

1 tablespoon lime juice

1 cup peeled, seeded, and roughly chopped cucumber

1 teaspoon stevia or your preferred low-calorie sweetener

1 cup ice

1. In a blender, combine the water, lime juice, cucumber, stevia, and ice and purée on medium speed until smooth, 60 to 90 seconds.

2. Pour into 2 glasses and enjoy.

3. Store any leftover smoothie in a sealed container, such as a mason jar with a lid, in the refrigerator for up to 2 days. The liquid and solid ingredients will separate and impact the taste and texture, so reblend the smoothie for 10 to 15 seconds before serving.

Variation tip: Add ½ teaspoon of alcohol-free vanilla extract if you prefer a less tart flavor profile.

Per Serving: Calories: 8.5gFat: 0.1g; Protein: 0.45g; Carbs: 2.74g; Fiber: 0.5g; Sugar: 1.18g; Sodium: 1.6mg

RASPBERRY REFRESHER

Prep time: 5 minutes   **Yield:** 3 (⅔-cup) servings

The just-picked sweet-tart flavors of raspberries blended with the subtly nutty taste of almond milk makes for a light and fruity treat. A touch of vanilla and pure maple syrup provides a sweet finish to this brisk berry blend that makes a great afternoon snack.

1 cup unsweetened almond milk

2 teaspoons alcohol-free vanilla extract

1 tablespoon plus 1 teaspoon pure maple syrup

1 cup fresh raspberries

1 cup ice

1. In a blender, combine the almond milk, vanilla, maple syrup, raspberries, and ice and purée on medium speed until smooth, 60 to 90 seconds.

2. Pour into glasses and enjoy.

3. Store any leftover smoothie in a sealed container, such as a mason jar with a lid, in the refrigerator for up to 2 days. The liquid and solid ingredients will separate and impact the taste and texture, so reblend the smoothie for 10 to 15 seconds before serving.

Variation tip: Mix a scoop of unflavored protein powder with the almond milk before blending to make this smoothie into a meal replacement shake.

Per Serving: Calories: 65.3; Fat: 1.1g; Protein: 0.84g; Carbs: 12.3g; Fiber: 2.8; Sugar: 8.1g; Sodium: 63.9mg

STRAWBERRY KIWI COOLER

Prep time: 5 minutes   **Yield:** 2 (1-cup) servings

Rich in vitamin C, strawberries and kiwi form the base for this rejuvenating drink. What could be better than a smoothie that provides a delicious alternative to plain water that will help you hydrate and inject a boost of refreshment into your day?

¾ cup almond milk

1 cup frozen strawberries

½ cup peeled and roughly chopped kiwi

1½ teaspoons stevia or your preferred low-calorie sweetener

1 cup ice

1. In a blender, combine the almond milk, strawberries, kiwi, stevia, and ice and purée on medium speed until smooth, about 90 seconds.

2. Pour into 2 glasses and enjoy.

3. Store any leftover smoothie in a sealed container, such as a mason jar with a lid, in the refrigerator for up to 2 days. The liquid and solid ingredients will separate and impact the taste and texture, so reblend the smoothie for 10 to 15 seconds before serving.

Prep tip: If you are less than 3 months post-bariatric surgery, you may have a hard time tolerating the kiwi seeds. Strain them from the smoothie using an extra-fine-mesh strainer. (Note that this will reduce the volume yield of the recipe slightly.)

Per Serving: Calories: 79.5; Fat: 1.1g; Protein: 1.1g; Carbs: 17.9g; Fiber: 3.1g; Sugar: 11.79g; Sodium: 66.7mg

POWER C SMOOTHIE

Prep time: 5 minutes   **Yield:** 2 (1-cup) servings

Boost your energy and immunity with just one dose of this delicious and tart drink. A blend of grapefruit, orange, lemon, and lime juices provides a tonic rich in vitamin C that you can enjoy any time of day.

2 tablespoons
   no-sugar-added
   grapefruit juice
2 tablespoons
   no-sugar-added
   orange juice
1 tablespoon
   lemon juice
1 tablespoon lime juice
2 teaspoons pure
   maple syrup
½ cup water
1 cup ice

1. In a blender, combine the grapefruit juice, orange juice, lemon juice, lime juice, maple syrup, water, and ice and purée on medium speed until smooth, about 30 seconds.

2. Pour into 2 glasses and enjoy.

3. Store any leftover smoothie in a sealed container, such as a mason jar with a lid, in the refrigerator for up to 2 days. The ingredients will separate and impact the taste and texture, so reblend the smoothie for 10 to 15 seconds before serving.

Post-op tip: In the later stages of your post-op journey, feel free to blend in the flesh of the citrus fruits for extra fiber.

Per Serving: Calories: 34.4; Fat: .06g; Protein: 0.27g; Carbs: 9.5g; Fiber: 0.14g; Sugar: 7.15g; Sodium: 1.65mg

CUCUMBER KIWI COOLER

Prep time: 5 minutes   **Yield:** 2 (1-cup) servings

This one is especially enjoyable on a hot day or as a post-workout hydration beverage. But no matter when you drink it, this smoothie is sure to please your taste buds with the complex fruitiness of kiwi and the soothing cucumber, which keeps things cool.

½ cup water

1 cup peeled, seeded, and roughly chopped cucumber

½ cup peeled and roughly chopped kiwi

2 teaspoons pure maple syrup

1 cup ice

1. In a blender, combine the water, cucumber, kiwi, maple syrup, and ice and purée on medium speed until smooth, about 60 seconds.

2. Pour into 2 glasses and enjoy.

3. Store any leftover smoothie in a sealed container, such as a mason jar with a lid, in the refrigerator for up to 2 days. The liquid and solid ingredients will separate and impact the taste and texture, so reblend the smoothie for 10 to 15 seconds before serving.

Post-op tip: Be sure to strain the kiwi seeds from the smoothie in an extra-fine-mesh strainer if consuming this drink before the 3-month mark of your post-op journey. (Note that this will reduce the volume yield of the recipe slightly.)

Per Serving: Calories: 50; Fat: 0.28g; Protein: 0.87g; Carbs: 12.2g; Fiber: 1.8g; Sugar: 9g; Sodium: 4.4mg

BLUE RASPBERRY REFRESHER

Prep time: 3 minutes   **Yield:** 2 (1-cup) servings

If you enjoy the taste of freezer pops and popsicles (and who doesn't?), you'll love this natural rendition with its tart and sweet berry flavors. This gorgeous, brightly colored smoothie is a delight for the eyes and the tummy and will keep you refreshed for hours.

¾ cup water

1 cup frozen blueberries

½ cup fresh raspberries

2 teaspoons pure
  maple syrup

1 cup ice

1. In a blender, combine the water, blueberries, raspberries, maple syrup, and ice and purée on medium speed until smooth, 60 to 90 seconds.

2. Pour into 2 glasses and enjoy.

3. Store any leftover smoothie in a sealed container, such as a mason jar with a lid, in the refrigerator for up to 2 days. The liquid and solid ingredients will separate and impact the taste and texture, so reblend the smoothie for 10 to 15 seconds before serving.

Prep tip: Feel free to substitute frozen raspberries if they are easier to come by than fresh, but you should omit the ice to maintain a pourable consistency. This will also result in a slightly lower yield of 2 (¾-cup) servings.

Per Serving: Calories: 73; Fat: 0.67g; Protein: .7g; Carbs: 17.5g; Fiber: 4g; Sugar: 11.9g; Sodium: 1.8mg

MOJITO-STYLE COCONUT LIME AND MINT COOLER

Prep time: 5 minutes   **Yield:** 1 (1¼-cup) serving

Alcohol is not recommended for the first six months post-op when you are healing, but you can still enjoy the refreshing flavors of a mojito in this low-carb, nonalcoholic cooler. You'll get the tropical vacation vibe you love along with the hydration you need.

½ cup almond milk

5 tablespoons canned unsweetened coconut milk

½ teaspoon alcohol-free vanilla extract

2 tablespoons lime juice

About 6 (1-inch) fresh mint leaves

2 teaspoons pure maple syrup

1 cup ice

1. In a blender, combine the almond milk, coconut milk, vanilla, lime juice, mint leaves, maple syrup, and ice and purée on medium speed until smooth, about 60 seconds.

2. Pour into a glass and enjoy.

Prep tip: Add a bit more alcohol-free vanilla extract if you prefer a smoother and sweeter flavor profile.

Per Serving: Calories: 99.5; Fat: 6.65g; Protein: 0.36g; Carbs: 11.8g; Fiber: 0.25g; Sugar: 7.5g; Sodium: 49.5mg

STRAWBERRY LIME REFRESHER

Prep time: 3 minutes   **Yield:** 2 (1¼-cup) servings

If you are a fan of the puckering sweetness of strawberry lemonade, this drink is for you. The citrus highlights the flavor of the berries, making it a classic combination for good reason. Feel free to add more lime juice or a bit of lemon juice for an extra-tart taste that is very appealing.

1 cup water

2 tablespoons lime juice

1 cup frozen strawberries

1 tablespoon plus 1 teaspoon pure maple syrup

1 cup ice

1. In a blender, combine the water, lime juice, strawberries, maple syrup, and ice and purée on medium speed until smooth, about 60 seconds.

2. Pour into 2 glasses and enjoy.

3. Store any leftover smoothie in a sealed container, such as a mason jar with a lid, in the refrigerator for up to 2 days. The liquid and solid ingredients will separate and impact the taste and texture, so reblend the smoothie for 10 to 15 seconds before serving.

Variation tip: To change things up, try substituting blackberries for the strawberries.

Per Serving: Calories: 55.8; Fat: 0.34g; Protein: 0.45g; Carbs: 16g; Fiber: 1.68g; Sugar: 9.9g; Sodium: 3.3mg

GREEN TEA LIME COOLER

Prep time: 1 hour 15 minutes   **Yield:** 2 (¾-cup) servings

For the ultimate in antioxidant refreshment, you can't go wrong with this tart tea-based beverage. The naturally bitter taste of green tea—a giveaway that it's an antioxidant powerhouse—paired with the bright flavor of lime juice provides a refreshing drink that will soothe your gut, plus it has a little caffeine kick that's a perfect pick-me-up for mornings or midafternoon slumps.

2 green tea bags

2 tablespoons lime juice

**1 tablespoon plus
  1 teaspoon pure
  maple syrup**

1 cup ice

1. Bring a kettle of water to a boil over high heat.

2. Place the tea bags in a heatproof mug and pour 1 cup of boiling water into the mug. Let steep for 10 minutes. Remove and discard the tea bags.

3. Chill the tea in the refrigerator for at least 1 hour.

4. In a blender, combine the brewed green tea, lime juice, maple syrup, and ice and purée until smooth, about 30 seconds.

5. Pour into 2 glasses and enjoy.

6. Store any leftover smoothie in a sealed container, such as a mason jar with a lid, in the refrigerator for up to 2 days. The ingredients will separate and impact the taste and texture, so reblend the smoothie for 10 to 15 seconds before serving.

Prep tip: To cut down on prep time, brew the tea ahead of time and store it in an airtight container in the refrigerator until ready to use.

Variation tip: Add ½ cup of unsweetened almond milk if you prefer a smoother, less tart flavor, though this will mellow out the flavors of the finished smoothie. It will also add a few calories.

Per Serving: Calories: 41; Fat: 0g; Protein: 0.33g; Carbs: 11.5g; Fiber: 0.1g; Sugar: 4.5g; Sodium: 4.6mg

BLUEBERRY LEMON COOLER

Prep time: 3 minutes   **Yield:** 2 (1-cup) servings

Here is another spin on the winning marriage of citrus and berries. In this appealing beverage, vitamin C and antioxidant-rich blueberries double down on the health benefits. This smoothie offers intense hydration and anti-inflammation properties. It's the ideal choice whenever you're feeling like you need a boost.

1 cup water

2 tablespoons lemon juice

1 tablespoon pure maple syrup

1 cup frozen blueberries

1. In a blender, combine the water, lemon juice, maple syrup, and blueberries and purée on medium speed until smooth, about 60 seconds.

2. Pour into 2 glasses and enjoy.

3. Store any leftover smoothie in a sealed container, such as a mason jar with a lid, in the refrigerator for up to 2 days. The liquid and solid ingredients will separate and impact the taste and texture, so reblend the smoothie for 10 to 15 seconds before serving.

Prep tip: If you don't have frozen blueberries on hand, feel free to use 1 cup of fresh blueberries and add ½ cup of ice. Keep in mind that using fresh blueberries instead of frozen will decrease the yield of the smoothie slightly.

Per Serving: Calories: 69; Fat: 0.5g; Protein: 0.37g; Carbs: 17.2 g; Fiber: 2.2g; Sugar: 12.9g; Sodium: 2.1mg

BLUEBERRY GREEN TEA REFRESHER

Prep time: 1 hour 15 minutes   **Yield:** 2 (1-cup) servings

Offset the naturally bitter taste of green tea with the subtly sweet and tart flavors of blueberries. This combination gives this satisfying beverage a smooth, mellow taste that's appealing either cool or warmed. To serve it warm, add the brewed green tea to the blender while it is still hot.

2 green tea bags

½ cup frozen blueberries

1 tablespoon plus 1 teaspoon pure maple syrup or honey

1 cup ice

1. Bring a kettle of water to a boil over high heat.

2. Place the tea bags in a heatproof mug and pour 1 cup of boiling water into the mug. Let steep for 10 minutes. Remove and discard the tea bags.

3. Chill the tea in the refrigerator for at least 1 hour.

4. In a blender, combine the chilled green tea, blueberries, maple syrup, and ice and purée on medium speed for about 60 seconds.

5. Pour into 2 glasses and enjoy.

6. Store any leftover smoothie in a sealed container, such as a mason jar with a lid, in the refrigerator for up to 2 days. The liquid and solid ingredients will separate and impact the taste and texture, so reblend the smoothie for 10 to 15 seconds before serving.

Prep tip: To cut down on prep time, brew the tea ahead of time and store it in an airtight container in the refrigerator until ready to use.

Variation tip: Add a teaspoon or two of lemon juice for an extra tart taste.

Per Serving: Calories: 57; Fat: 0.5g; Protein: 0.7g; Carbs: 13.6g; Fiber: 2g; Sugar: 11.25g; Sodium: 4.4mg

STRAWBERRY CITRUS GREEN TEA

Prep time: 1 hour 15 minutes   **Yield:** 1 (1¼-cup) serving

Sweeten up your green tea with a blend of strawberries and give it a touch of brightness with a little lemon juice. Filled with healing antioxidants, this tea-based smoothie is soothing and delicious while it hydrates your recovering tummy.

2 green tea bags

1 tablespoon lemon juice

1 cup frozen strawberries

1 tablespoon pure maple syrup or honey

1. Bring a kettle of water to a boil over high heat.

2. Place the tea bags in a heatproof mug and pour ¾ cup of boiling water into the mug. Let steep for 10 minutes. Remove and discard the tea bags.

3. Chill the tea in the refrigerator for at least 1 hour.

4. In a blender, combine the chilled green tea, lemon juice, strawberries, and maple syrup and purée on medium speed until smooth, about 60 seconds.

5. Pour into a glass and enjoy.

Post-op tip: If you have trouble tolerating seeds, strain the seeds using a fine-mesh strainer.

Prep tip: To cut down on prep time, brew the tea ahead of time and store it in an airtight container in the refrigerator until ready to use.

Per Serving: Calories: 56; Fat: 0.1g; Protein: 0.88g; Carbs: 14g; Fiber: 1.5g; Sugar: 8.1g; Sodium: 5.2mg

PEACH ALMOND MILK REFRESHER

Prep time: 3 minutes   **Yield:** 2 (¾-cup) servings

The mild peaches-and-cream flavor of this refresher has a pleasing, gentle sweetness that's just what you need while you recover. Try this one if you're in the mood for something that's easy on the taste buds but still flavorful.

1 cup almond milk

¾ cup frozen peaches

2 teaspoons pure maple syrup

1. In a blender, combine the almond milk, peaches, and maple syrup and purée on medium speed until smooth, about 30 seconds.

2. Pour into 2 glasses and enjoy.

3. Store any leftover smoothie in a sealed container, such as a mason jar with a lid, in the refrigerator for up to 2 days. The liquid and solid ingredients will separate and impact the taste and texture, so reblend the smoothie for 10 to 15 seconds before serving.

Variation tip: Add more frozen peaches, if you like, to enhance the peach flavor, but keep in mind that this will increase the sugar content, the caloric content, and the volume of the drink.

Per Serving: Calories: 79; Fat: 1.5g; Protein: 1.0g; Carbs: 16.5g; Fiber: 1.5g; Sugar: 15g; Sodium: 76mg

BLUEBERRY GRAPEFRUIT COOLER

Prep time: 3 minutes   **Yield:** 2 (1-cup) servings

Usually reserved for breakfast buffets and cocktails, grapefruit seems like an under-rated citrus juice. Its slight bitterness is not for everyone, but if that's not a concern, I highly recommend that you try this recipe. Please note that some medications may interact with grapefruit, so be sure to check with your doctor before adding it to your smoothies. If you can't have grapefruit, omit it and use the same amount of orange juice for a similar flavor.

1 cup fresh or frozen blueberries

½ cup no-sugar-added grapefruit juice

1 tablespoon pure maple syrup

1 cup ice

1. In a blender, combine the blueberries, grapefruit juice, maple syrup, and ice and purée on medium speed until smooth, about 60 seconds.

2. Pour into 2 glasses and enjoy.

3. Store any leftover smoothie in a sealed container, such as a mason jar with a lid, in the refrigerator for up to 2 days. The liquid and solid ingredients will separate and impact the taste and texture, so reblend the smoothie for 10 to 15 seconds before serving.

Prep tip: Add ¼ teaspoon of minced fresh ginger for a slightly spicy flavor and as an extra boost to support gut health.

Variation tip: If you choose frozen blueberries instead of fresh, remember to reduce or omit the ice entirely to keep the smoothie pourable, and note that the yield of the recipe will be slightly lower.

Per Serving: Calories: 59; Fat: 0.4g; Protein: 0.4; Carbs: 14.5; Fiber: 1.46g; Sugar: 12.1g; Sodium: 1.46mg

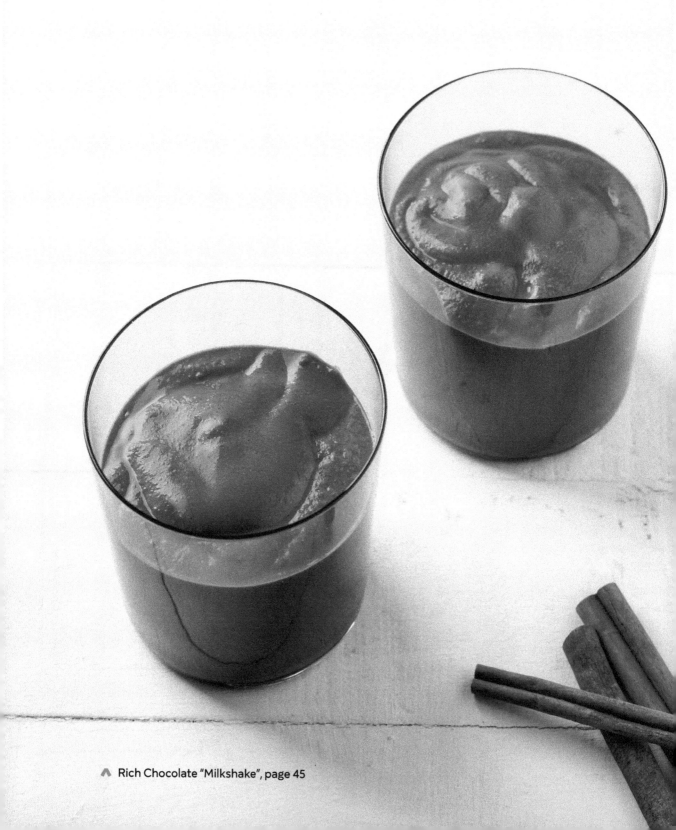

Rich Chocolate "Milkshake", page 45

3

CREAMY

The recipes in this chapter take advantage of the luxurious and satisfying textures that you can only create in smoothies by adding dairy, nondairy milks, or coconut cream. These creamy, delicious smoothies are sweet and decadent enough to stand in as a dessert alternative or a simple snack when your sweet tooth comes calling. Some of them are thick enough to be enjoyed with a spoon.

Many of them include good sources of protein, but feel free to add more in the form of your favorite protein powder, milk, or plant-based milk product. After drinking one of these smoothies, you won't miss that slice of cake or scoop of ice cream you may have been craving.

COCONUT VANILLA CREAM SMOOTHIE

Prep time: 5 minutes　**Yield:** 2 (½-cup) servings

The flavor of coconut is so closely associated with the tropics, it's hard not to feel like you're on vacation when drinking this decadent smoothie. It's a delicious alternative if you're craving a creamy dessert or just want to feel like you are miles away. When using canned coconut milk, use a butter knife to slowly stir together the liquids and solids well before measuring it and adding it to the blender.

½ cup plain nonfat Greek yogurt

½ cup canned unsweetened coconut milk

1 tablespoon alcohol-free vanilla extract

2 teaspoons stevia or your favorite low-calorie sweetener

½ cup ice

1. In a blender, combine the yogurt, coconut milk, vanilla, stevia, and ice and purée on medium speed until smooth, 60 to 90 seconds.

2. Pour into 2 glasses and enjoy.

3. Store any leftover smoothie in a sealed container, such as a mason jar with a lid, in the refrigerator for up to 2 days. The liquid and solid ingredients will separate and impact the taste and texture, so reblend the smoothie for 10 to 15 seconds before serving.

Prep tip: For an extra kick of coconut flavor, add ¼ teaspoon of coconut extract (or to taste) to the mix.

Per Serving: Calories: 145; Fat: 10g; Protein: 6.3g; Carbs: 6g; Fiber: .45g; Sugar: 3.5g; Sodium: 33.8mg

PUMPKIN NUT SMOOTHIE

Prep time: 5 minutes   **Yield:** 2 (¾-cup) servings

If you love the creamy taste of peanut butter, then you'll love this fiber- and antioxidant-rich smoothie blend that is reminiscent of a more decadent peanut butter milkshake. The puréed pumpkin provides a smooth and thick consistency. Try adding a touch of your favorite sweetener to make it feel even more indulgent.

1 cup soy milk

1 cup unsweetened pumpkin purée

2 tablespoons unsweetened creamy peanut butter

¼ cup peeled and chopped apple

1. In a blender, combine the soy milk, pumpkin purée, peanut butter, and apple and purée on medium speed for 30 to 60 seconds.

2. Pour into 2 glasses and enjoy.

3. Store any leftover smoothie in a sealed container, such as a mason jar with a lid, in the refrigerator for up to 2 days. The liquid and solid ingredients will separate and impact the taste and texture, so reblend the smoothie for 10 to 15 seconds before serving.

Post-op tip: Mix a little vanilla-flavored, low-sugar protein powder with the soy milk before adding to the blender for a boost of sweetness and protein without impacting the intended flavor profile too much. You may have to add a bit more soy milk to reach the consistency you want and to avoid grittiness, which will increase the calories a bit.

Per Serving: Calories: 150; Fat: 6g; Protein: 5.6g; Carbs: 13.3g; Fiber: 3.2g; Sugar: 6.8g; Sodium: 89mg

LEMON CREAM PIE COOLER

Prep time: 5 minutes   **Yield:** 2 (½-cup) servings

If you love lemon, I'm sure you'll agree that in this smoothie, tart and sweet blend together perfectly, making it reminiscent of a lemon cream pie. Thick and creamy, just a small glass will satisfy your dessert cravings due to its rich protein content and flavor. I suggest you eat this with a spoon to complete the illusion.

½ cup canned unsweet- ened coconut milk

½ cup plain nonfat Greek yogurt

1 teaspoon freshly squeezed lemon juice

¼ teaspoon lemon zest

1½ teaspoons stevia or your preferred low-calorie sweetener

1 teaspoon alcohol-free vanilla extract

½ cup ice

1. In a blender, combine the coconut milk, yogurt, lemon juice, lemon zest, stevia, vanilla, and ice and purée on low speed until smooth, about 60 seconds.

2. Pour into 2 glasses and enjoy.

3. Store any leftover smoothie in a sealed container, such as a mason jar with a lid, in the refrigerator for up to 2 days. The liquid and solid ingredients will separate and impact the taste and texture, so reblend the smoothie for 10 to 15 seconds before serving.

Variation tip: Use lime juice and lime zest instead of lemon to create a Key lime pie–like smoothie.

Per Serving: Calories: 134; Fat: 10.2g; Protein: 6.3g; Carbs: 4.2g; Fiber: 0g; Sugar: 3.1g; Sodium: 33.5mg

BLUEBERRY COMPOTE COOLER

Prep time: 5 minutes   **Yield:** 2 (½-cup) servings

Savor the nostalgic flavors of fresh blueberry crisp with this smooth and creamy blueberry smoothie. A handful of quick-cooked oats gives it an extra-thick texture while adding a bit of fiber that will help support your gut health.

2 tablespoons quick (1-minute) oats

2 tablespoons hot water

½ cup almond milk, at room temperature

1 cup frozen blueberries

1 teaspoon honey or brown sugar

1. In a small bowl, mix together the quick oats, hot water, and almond milk and let sit until the oats are rehydrated and thickened, 1 to 2 minutes.

2. In a blender, combine the oat mixture, blueberries, and honey and purée on high speed until smooth, 60 to 90 seconds.

3. Pour into 2 glasses and enjoy.

4. Store any leftover smoothie in a sealed container, such as a mason jar with a lid, in the refrigerator for up to 2 days. The liquid and solid ingredients will separate and impact the taste and texture, so reblend the smoothie for 10 to 15 seconds before serving.

Prep tip: Add 1 to 2 tablespoons of buttermilk to give this smoothie an unexpected and delightful buttery crust flavor—just like your favorite crisp. Just be aware that it will add a few calories to the beverage.

Per Serving: Calories: 77; Fat: 1.3g; Protein: 1.26g; Carbs: 11.9g; Fiber: 2.46g; Sugar: 11.7g; Sodium: 44mg

DARK CHOCOLATE-COVERED STRAWBERRY SMOOTHIE

Prep time: 3 minutes   **Yield:** 2 (½-cup) servings

Chocolate and fruit are a classic combination that tastes great in liquid form. One sip of this smoothie will have you thinking you're indulging in a guilty pleasure.

1 cup unsweetened almond milk

1 cup frozen strawberries

2 tablespoons unsweetened cocoa powder

1. In a blender, combine the almond milk, strawberries, and cocoa powder and purée on high speed until smooth, about 60 seconds.

2. Pour into 2 glasses and enjoy.

3. Store any leftover smoothie in a sealed container, such as a mason jar with a lid, in the refrigerator for up to 2 days. The liquid and solid ingredients will separate and impact the taste and texture, so reblend the smoothie for 10 to 15 seconds before serving.

Prep tip: Add a few tablespoons of coconut milk for extra-creamy flavor or 1 teaspoon of honey or your favorite low-calorie sweetener for extra sweetness. Coconut milk and honey will add a few calories to the drink.

Per Serving: Calories: 58; Fat: 2.1g; Protein: 1.9g; Carbs: 11.6g; Fiber: 3.8g; Sugar: 4.5g; Sodium: 96.5mg

STRAWBERRY CHEESECAKE SMOOTHIE

Prep time: 5 minutes   **Yield:** 2 (¾-cup) servings

If you love cheesecake but are post-op and can't tolerate the sugar and fat content of such desserts, look no further. The tang of cottage cheese and buttermilk mimics the flavors of cheesecake and gives this smoothie added protein to boot. The strawberries bring a fruity sweetness.

¾ cup **4 percent milkfat cottage cheese**

2 teaspoons alcohol-free vanilla extract

⅓ **cup unsweetened almond milk**

⅓ **cup low-fat buttermilk**

1 cup frozen strawberries

2 teaspoons stevia or your preferred low-calorie sweetener

1. In a blender, combine the cottage cheese, vanilla, almond milk, buttermilk, strawberries, and stevia and purée on high speed until smooth, about 60 seconds.

2. Pour into 2 glasses and enjoy.

3. Store any leftover smoothie in a sealed container, such as a mason jar with a lid, in the refrigerator for up to 2 days. The liquid and solid ingredients will separate and impact the taste and texture, so reblend the smoothie for 10 to 15 seconds before serving.

Post-op tip: If you are having trouble tolerating any small amount of fat, try using a lower-fat cottage cheese in this recipe, which will actually lower the calories a bit. If you are lactose intolerant, look for a lactose-free variety.

Per Serving: Calories: 138.5; Fat: 4.3g; Protein: 10.6g; Carbs: 12.5g; Fiber: 1.6g; Sugar: 9.8g; Sodium: 342mg

PEANUT BUTTER AND STRAWBERRY JAM SMOOTHIE

Prep time: 5 minutes   **Yield:** 2 (½-cup) servings

The simple and delicious flavor combination of peanut butter and jam is a comforting classic. It translates beautifully from your childhood sandwich to this nutty smoothie, which gets its extra nutrition from the protein-packed peanut butter.

½ **cup almond milk**

1 **teaspoon alcohol-free vanilla extract**

¼ **cup canned unsweetened coconut milk**

1 **tablespoon peanut butter**

½ **cup frozen strawberries**

1. In a blender, combine the almond milk, vanilla, coconut milk, peanut butter, and strawberries and purée on high speed until smooth, about 60 seconds.

2. Pour into 2 glasses and enjoy.

3. Store any leftover smoothie in a sealed container, such as a mason jar with a lid, in the refrigerator for up to 2 days. The liquid and solid ingredients will separate and impact the taste and texture, so reblend the smoothie for 10 to 15 seconds before serving.

Prep tip: Try mixing a scoop of your favorite unflavored or vanilla-flavored, low-sugar protein powder with the almond milk before blending to make this into a meal replacement shake. Keep in mind that you may have to add a bit more almond milk to get the consistency you want, which will raise the calories a bit.

Per Serving: Calories: 131; Fat: 9.8g; Protein: 2.35g; Carbs: 9g; Fiber: 1.4g; Sugar: 5.5g; Sodium: 77mg

RICH CHOCOLATE "MILKSHAKE"

Prep time: 5 minutes   **Yield:** 2 (½-cup) servings

When you're not yet ready to eat solids, especially the high-sugar kind, this shake can be a great alternative to satisfy any craving you might have for a chocolate bar. With bold chocolate flavor and caramel notes from coconut, this is a smoothie your taste buds won't soon forget. To kick it up another notch, try adding a pinch of ground cinnamon.

½ cup almond milk

¼ cup canned unsweetened coconut milk

1 tablespoon pure maple syrup

1 teaspoon alcohol-free vanilla extract

1 tablespoon unsweetened cocoa powder

½ cup ice

1. In a blender, combine the almond milk, coconut milk, maple syrup, vanilla, cocoa powder, and ice and purée on low speed until smooth, about 60 seconds.

2. Pour into 2 glasses and enjoy.

3. Store any leftover smoothie in a sealed container, such as a mason jar with a lid, in the refrigerator for up to 2 days. The liquid and solid ingredients will separate and impact the taste and texture, so reblend the smoothie for 10 to 15 seconds before serving.

Prep tip: If you prefer a creamier texture, you can add more unsweetened coconut milk and/or reduce the amount of ice. If you add more coconut milk, take note that the smoothie will be less sweet, and you may want to add more maple syrup, which will add more carbohydrates to the recipe. Another alternative is to add 1 teaspoon of your favorite low-calorie sweetener.

Per Serving: Calories: 101; Fat: 5.8g; Protein: .76g; Carbs: 12.5g; Fiber: 1.1g; Sugar: 9.6g; Sodium: 49.5mg

PEANUT BUTTER CHOCOLATE CUP SMOOTHIE

Prep time: 5 minutes   **Yield:** 2 (¾-cup) servings

There's nothing like the combination of peanut butter and chocolate to make you feel like you're indulging in a favorite childhood treat. The best part about this smoothie is that it's low in carbohydrates while still being full of natural antioxidants from the cocoa powder. Add more maple syrup or your preferred sweetener if you'd like a sweeter smoothie.

½ cup canned unsweet-
ened coconut milk

½ cup almond milk

2 tablespoons unsweet-
ened cocoa powder

2 tablespoons creamy
peanut butter

1 tablespoon
plus 1 teaspoon
alcohol-free
vanilla extract

2 teaspoons pure
maple syrup

1. In a blender, combine the coconut milk, almond milk, cocoa powder, peanut butter, vanilla, and maple syrup and purée on low speed until smooth. about 30 seconds.

2. Pour into 2 glasses and enjoy.

3. Store any leftover smoothie in a sealed container, such as a mason jar with a lid, in the refrigerator for up to 2 days. The liquid and solid ingredients will separate and impact the taste and texture, so reblend the smoothie for 10 to 15 seconds before serving.

Post-op tip: If you want this shake to be a meal replacement, mix 1 scoop of your favorite unflavored, chocolate-, or peanut butter–flavored, low-sugar protein powder with the almond milk before adding to the blender.

Prep tip: If you prefer, you can use the same amount of powdered peanut butter instead of natural peanut butter. The protein content will be about the same, but the powdered peanut butter will have about one-third of the calories and much less fat.

Per Serving: Calories: 259; Fat: 19.7g; Protein: 5.2g; Carbs: 16g; Fiber: 3.1g; Sugar: 9.2g; Sodium: 113mg

MINT CHOCOLATE COOLER

Prep time: 5 minutes   **Yield:** 2 (½-cup) servings

Thin mint candy lovers, head to the front of the class! The cool, refreshing flavor of mint and the creamy, rich flavor of chocolate go just as well together in this smoothie as they do in everyone's favorite peppermint patties.

1 cup canned unsweet-ened coconut milk

2 teaspoons unsweet-ened cocoa powder

2 teaspoons alcohol-free vanilla extract

About 6 (1-inch) fresh mint leaves

¼ teaspoon pepper-mint extract

1 tablespoon plus 1 teaspoon pure maple syrup

1. In a blender, combine the coconut milk, cocoa powder, vanilla, mint leaves, peppermint extract, and maple syrup and purée on low speed until smooth, about 30 seconds.

2. Pour into 2 glasses and enjoy.

3. Store any leftover smoothie in a sealed container, such as a mason jar with a lid, in the refrigerator for up to 2 days. The liquid and solid ingredients will separate and impact the taste and texture, so reblend the smoothie for 10 to 15 seconds before serving.

Prep tip: Add more peppermint extract or mint leaves if you prefer a more intense taste, but be aware that a little goes a long way when it comes to peppermint flavor. You can also use a few drops of food-grade peppermint oil in lieu of peppermint extract if you prefer, but add it one drop at a time and blend after each addition until it reaches the flavor you want.

Per Serving: Calories: 232; Fat: 19.8g; Protein: 0.35g; Carbs: 14g; Fiber: 1.3g; Sugar: 13g; Sodium: 31mg

CINNAMON COCONUT COOLER

Prep time: 5 minutes   **Yield:** 2 (¾-cup) servings

Here is a spicy and smooth cooler that mimics the taste of horchata, the Mexican rice-based beverage. And like horchata, the texture is thinner than some of the other smoothies, but what it lacks in thickness it makes up for in rich, subtly sweet flavor.

½ cup unsweetened almond milk

½ cup canned unsweetened coconut milk

1 tablespoon alcohol-free vanilla extract

1 teaspoon ground cinnamon

1 teaspoon pure maple syrup

½ cup ice

1. In a blender, combine the almond milk, coconut milk, vanilla, cinnamon, maple syrup, and ice and purée on low speed until smooth, about 30 seconds.

2. Pour into 2 glasses and enjoy.

3. Store any leftover smoothie in a sealed container, such as a mason jar with a lid, in the refrigerator for up to 2 days. The liquid and solid ingredients will separate and impact the taste and texture, so reblend the smoothie for 10 to 15 seconds before serving.

Prep tip: For a creamier texture, omit the ice, but keep in mind that it will affect the yield of the recipe.

Per Serving: Calories: 138; Fat: 10.3g; Protein: 0.3g; Carbs: 8.8g; Fiber: 0.8g; Sugar: 6.5g; Sodium: 54mg

PUMPKIN PIE SMOOTHIE

Prep time: 5 minutes   **Yield:** 2 (½-cup) servings

Biting into a forkful of pumpkin pie topped with a dollop of whipped cream evokes cozy and comforting feelings, but you don't need to relegate it to the fall and winter holiday seasons. This low-sugar smoothie lets you enjoy the fresh and creamy flavors of pumpkin pie any time you want.

½ cup unsweetened pumpkin purée

½ cup canned unsweetened coconut milk

2 tablespoons plain nonfat Greek yogurt

2 teaspoons alcohol-free vanilla extract

1 teaspoon ground cinnamon

1 tablespoon plus 1 teaspoon pure maple syrup or your preferred sweetener

½ cup ice

1. In a blender, combine the pumpkin purée, coconut milk, yogurt, vanilla, cinnamon, maple syrup, and ice and purée on low speed until smooth, about 60 seconds.

2. Pour into 2 glasses and enjoy.

3. Store any leftover smoothie in a sealed container, such as a mason jar with a lid, in the refrigerator for up to 2 days. The liquid and solid ingredients will separate and impact the taste and texture, so reblend the smoothie for 10 to 15 seconds before serving.

Variation tip: Omit the cinnamon and add 1 teaspoon of pumpkin pie spice to get an extra depth of pumpkin pie flavor.

Per Serving: Calories: 171; Fat: 11.7g; Protein: 2.3g; Carbs: 17.3g; Fiber: 2.4g; Sugar: 13.3g; Sodium: 28mg

PEACHES AND CREAM SMOOTHIE

Prep time: 3 minutes   **Yield:** 1 (¾-cup) smoothie

This is a filling smoothie, thanks to the coconut milk, which goes nicely with the subtle flavor of peaches. Your recovering gut will thank you.

½ cup canned unsweet-
  ened coconut milk

½ cup frozen peaches

1 teaspoon alcohol-free
  vanilla extract

2 teaspoons pure
  maple syrup

1. In a blender, combine the coconut milk, peaches, vanilla, and maple syrup and purée on low speed until smooth, about 60 seconds.

2. Pour into a glass and enjoy.

Post-op tip: Add more peaches as desired to amp up the peachy flavor, but keep in mind that this will increase the sugar content, the caloric content, and the volume of the drink.

Per Serving: Calories: 246; Fat: 19.7g; Protein: 0.7g; Carbs: 15.5g; Fiber: 1.1g; Sugar: 12.3g; Sodium: 33.6mg

ORANGE CREAM SMOOTHIE

Prep time: 5 minutes   **Yield:** 1 (¾-cup) serving

Inspired by the dreamy taste of orange cream popsicles, this refreshing beverage will remind you of carefree childhood summers. You can even pour it into popsicle molds and freeze them to complete that feeling of nostalgia.

¼ **cup canned unsweet-
ened coconut milk**

¼ **cup plain nonfat
Greek yogurt**

¼ **teaspoon orange zest**

¼ **cup freshly squeezed
orange juice**

1 **teaspoon alcohol-free
vanilla extract**

1 **teaspoon stevia
or your preferred
low-calorie sweetener**

½ **cup ice (optional)**

1. In a blender, combine the coconut milk, yogurt, orange zest, orange juice, vanilla, stevia, and ice (if using) and purée on low speed until smooth, about 30 seconds.

2. Pour into a glass and enjoy.

Post-op tip: When you have recovered enough to tolerate solid fibers from produce, try adding a few orange slices, including the peel, to the blender instead of orange juice for an extra hit of citrus flavor.

Per Serving: Calories: 169; Fat: 10g; Protein: 6.6g; Carbs: 11.3g; Fiber: 0.74g; Sugar: 8.4g; Sodium: 35mg

PINEAPPLE COCONUT COOLER

Prep time: 3 minutes   **Yield:** 1 (¾-cup) serving

What's not to like about piña coladas? Coconut, pineapple, and a dash of vanilla are a wonderful combination that can't be beat. And it's a great choice when you are recovering from surgery because it will soothe your stomach and satisfy your need for fabulous flavor. Add the ice for an extra-refreshing experience.

½ cup canned unsweet-
   ened coconut milk

½ cup unsweetened
   pineapple juice

1 teaspoon alcohol-free
   vanilla extract

½ cup ice (optional)

1. In a blender, combine the coconut milk, pineapple juice, vanilla, and ice (if using) and purée on low speed until smooth, 15 to 30 seconds.

2. Pour into a glass and enjoy.

Post-op tip: Once you recover enough to tolerate fibrous produce, omit the pineapple juice and add ½ cup of fresh or frozen diced pineapple instead for more fiber and extra pineapple flavor.

Per Serving: Calories: 240; Fat: 19.5g; Protein: 0.3g; Carbs: 15.6g; Fiber: <1g; Sugar: 13g; Sodium: 24mg

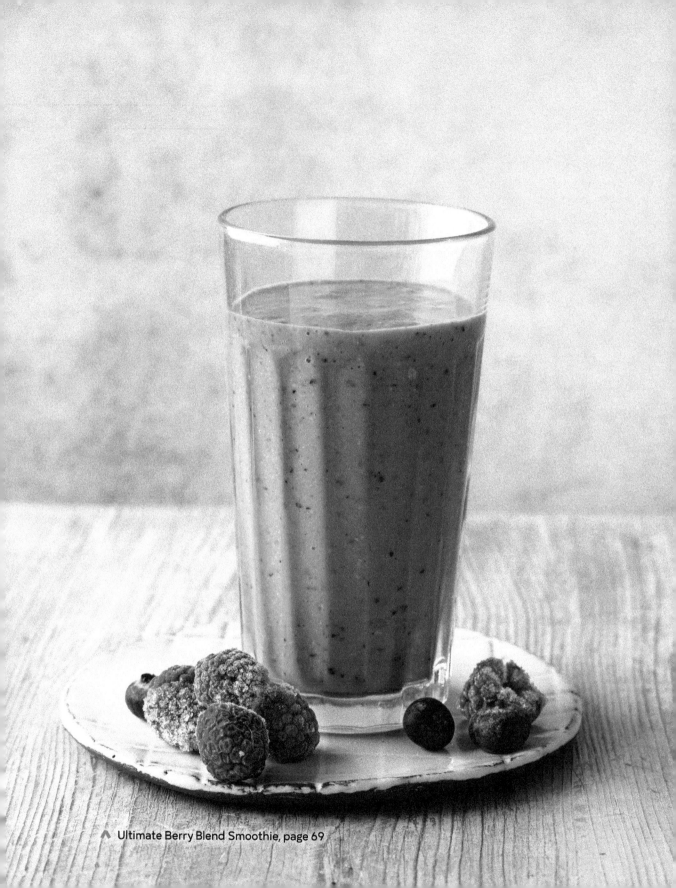

Ultimate Berry Blend Smoothie, page 69

4
FRUITY

Enjoy natural sweetness in every sip of these delicious and nutritious fiber- and antioxidant-rich recipes. Except for the clear liquids phase right after surgery, these work well for all post-op phases. The added fiber can help support your gut health as your digestive system heals.

STRAWBERRY COLADA COOLER

Prep time: 5 minutes   **Yield:** 2 (¾-cup) servings

This refreshingly tart smoothie is the perfect drink to enjoy outside on a warm day, but it's so hydrating and delicious, you should make it any time of year. You can use frozen berries from the supermarket or, even better, stock up on fresh when they're in season and freeze them for later use in recipes just like this one. Get out a spoon—this smoothie is extra thick and can double as a healthy dessert.

¾ cup unsweetened almond milk

2 tablespoons canned unsweetened coconut milk

2 teaspoons lime juice

1 teaspoon lemon juice

1 cup frozen strawberries

1. In a blender, combine the almond milk, coconut milk, lime juice, lemon juice, and strawberries and purée on medium speed until smooth, about 60 seconds.

2. Pour into 2 glasses and enjoy.

3. Store any leftover smoothie in a sealed container, such as a mason jar with a lid, in the refrigerator for up to 2 days. The liquid and solid ingredients will separate and impact the taste and texture, so reblend the smoothie for 10 to 15 seconds before serving.

Post-op tip: Mix some protein powder with the almond milk before adding to the blender if you prefer a higher-protein smoothie.

Variation tip: To increase the sweetness, add 1 teaspoon of your favorite low-calorie sweetener.

Per Serving: Calories: 77; Fat: 3.4g; Protein: 0.8g; Carbs: 13g; Fiber: 2.2g; Sugar: 8.1g; Sodium: 68mg

MANGO PEACH PINEAPPLE SMOOTHIE

Prep time: 3 minutes   **Yield:** 2 (½-cup) servings

Let the sunshine in with this tropical smoothie. The combination of almond milk and fruit juice may sound unusual, but it's mellow and delicious. Lower the liquid a bit and eat this as a sorbet, if you prefer.

¼ cup unsweetened almond milk

¼ cup unsweetened pineapple juice

½ cup frozen diced mango

½ cup frozen peach slices

1. In a blender, combine the almond milk, pineapple juice, mango, and peaches and purée on medium speed until smooth; about 60 seconds.

2. Pour into 2 glasses and enjoy.

3. Store any leftover smoothie in a sealed container, such as a mason jar with a lid, in the refrigerator for up to 2 days. The liquid and solid ingredients will separate and impact the taste and texture, so reblend the smoothie for 10 to 15 seconds before serving.

Prep tip: For a sweeter taste, feel free to add ¼ cup of peeled and chopped apples or a few more tablespoons of pineapple juice. However, take note that this will increase the sugar content, the caloric content, and the volume of the drink.

Variation tip: Substitute additional peaches for the mango if you don't like the taste or don't have access to it. Peaches are slightly lower in carbohydrates, which is also a bonus if you are looking for lower-carb recipes.

Per Serving: Calories: 60; Fat: 0.56g; Protein: .86g; Carbs: 10.7g; Fiber: 1.3g; Sugar: 11.7g; Sodium: 29.4mg

CHERRY BERRY LIME SMOOTHIE

Prep time: 5 minutes   **Yield:** 1 (¾-cup) serving

Here is a smoothie that may remind you of a sour candy treat, but I can assure you that this drink is low in sugar and provides antioxidant nutrition with each sip. And the texture is thick enough eat with a spoon like sorbet, if you prefer.

½ cup frozen
  strawberries
½ cup frozen pitted
  cherries
¼ cup water
1 teaspoon lime juice
1½ teaspoons stevia
  or your preferred
  low-calorie sweetener

1. In a blender, combine the strawberries, cherries, water, lime juice, and stevia and purée on high speed until smooth, about 45 seconds.

2. Pour into a glass and enjoy.

Prep tip: If you want to add protein and reduce the tartness of this recipe, add ¼ cup of plain nonfat Greek yogurt or mix 1 to 2 tablespoons of low-sugar protein powder with the water before blending.

Per Serving: Calories: 43; Fat: 0.1g; Protein: 0.5g; Carbs: 10.5g; Fiber: 2g; Sugar: 6.75g; Sodium: 1mg

BLUEBERRY COCONUT COOLER

Prep time: 3 minutes   **Yield:** 2 (¾-cup) servings

Combine antioxidant-rich blueberries and the subtle tropical flavor of coconut milk and you have a smoothie perfect for healing your gut. The subtly sweet and tart beverage is sure to please.

¾ cup unsweetened almond milk

½ cup canned unsweetened coconut milk

1 teaspoon alcohol-free vanilla extract

1 cup frozen blueberries

1. In a blender, combine the almond milk, coconut milk, vanilla, and blueberries and purée on medium speed until smooth, about 60 seconds.

2. Pour into 2 glasses and enjoy.

3. Store any leftover smoothie in a sealed container, such as a mason jar with a lid, in the refrigerator for up to 2 days. The liquid and solid ingredients will separate and impact the taste and texture, so reblend the smoothie for 10 to 15 seconds before serving.

Prep tip: For those less than 3 months post-op bariatric surgery, it may help to strain the smoothie through an extra-fine-mesh strainer to remove any excess blueberry skins before drinking to avoid possible gut irritation.

Per Serving: Calories: 163; Fat: 11.6g; Protein: 0.51g; Carbs: 16g; Fiber: 1.2g; Sugar: 8.6g; Sodium: 75mg

SIMPLE CANTALOUPE SMOOTHIE

Prep time: 5 minutes   **Yield:** 2 (1-cup) servings

The heady, floral flavor of ripe melon is a sensory treat that goes surprisingly well with tart yogurt in this smoothie, which is low in calories and carbohydrates. Melon also has a good amount of fiber with around 1½ grams for a cup of diced cantaloupe, for example. And cantaloupe contains the antioxidant lycopene, which is ideal for helping your body heal.

½ cup plain nonfat
  Greek yogurt
1¾ cups diced
  cantaloupe
1 teaspoon alcohol-free
  vanilla extract
1 cup ice

1. In a blender, combine the yogurt, cantaloupe, vanilla, and ice and purée on low speed until smooth, about 30 seconds.

2. Pour into 2 glasses and enjoy.

3. Store any leftover smoothie in a sealed container, such as a mason jar with a lid, in the refrigerator for up to 2 days. The liquid and solid ingredients will separate and impact the taste and texture, so reblend the smoothie for 10 to 15 seconds before serving.

Post-op tip: If you want to boost the vanilla flavor while adding protein, add your favorite brand of vanilla protein powder, a tablespoon at a time, to make sure the powder mixes in completely and the smoothie has a pourable consistency.

Per Serving: Calories: 90; Fat: 0.47g; Protein: 7.4g; Carbs: 13.5g; Fiber: 1.1g; Sugar: 13g; Sodium: 63mg

STRAWBERRY BANANA ORANGE SMOOTHIE

Prep time: 5 minutes **Yield:** 2 (¾-cup) servings

Smooth and sweet banana is the perfect foil for bright and sweet strawberries, making it a favorite combination for a reason. Here, the pair is joined by citrusy orange juice and zest for a trifecta of fruit flavors. Intentionally thick in texture, this smoothie is a great option for a meal alternative if you're still not ready for solids.

½ cup unsweetened almond milk

¼ teaspoon orange zest

2 tablespoons freshly squeezed orange juice

1 cup frozen strawberries

½ cup sliced bananas

1. In a blender, combine the almond milk, orange zest, orange juice, strawberries, and bananas and purée on medium speed until smooth, about 60 seconds.

2. Pour into 2 glasses and enjoy.

3. Store any leftover smoothie in a sealed container, such as a mason jar with a lid, in the refrigerator for up to 2 days. The liquid and solid ingredients will separate and impact the taste and texture, so reblend the smoothie for 10 to 15 seconds before serving.

Prep tip: To zest an orange, first wash the fruit. Using a cheese grater, remove the orange rind, making sure to avoid the bitter white pith. Wrap up any leftover zest for later use and refrigerate for up to 1 week.

Variation tip: Add 1 teaspoon of your preferred low-calorie sweetener or use slightly sweetened almond milk instead of unsweetened for an extra-sweet flavor. Sweetened almond milk will increase the sugar content and the caloric content of the drink.

Per Serving: Calories: 75; Fat: 1g; Protein: 1g; Carbs: 17g; Fiber: 2.75g; Sugar: 10.5g; Sodium: 28mg

BANANA MIXED BERRY SMOOTHIE

Prep time: 5 minutes   **Yield:** 2 (¾-cup) servings

With a blend of antioxidants from raspberries and blackberries and potassium and fiber from all the fruit, plus a bit of protein from the yogurt, this smoothie will put you quickly on the road to recovery.

½ cup unsweetened almond milk

½ cup plain nonfat Greek yogurt

½ cup sliced banana

½ cup frozen blackberries

½ cup frozen raspberries

½ cup ice

1 teaspoon stevia or your preferred low-calorie sweetener (optional)

1. In a blender, combine the almond milk, yogurt, banana, blackberries, raspberries, ice, and stevia (if using) and purée on medium speed until smooth, about 60 seconds.

2. Pour into 2 glasses and enjoy.

3. Store any leftover smoothie in a sealed container, such as a mason jar with a lid, in the refrigerator for up to 2 days. The liquid and solid ingredients will separate and impact the taste and texture, so reblend the smoothie for 10 to 15 seconds before serving.

Prep tip: You can use fresh berries instead of frozen, but be aware that you may require a bit more ice to create a thicker smoothie.

Per Serving: Calories: 79; Fat: 1g; Protein: 5.3g; Carbs: 14.3g; Fiber: 3g; Sugar: .675g; Sodium: 33.3mg

RASPBERRY PLUM SMOOTHIE

Prep time: 5 minutes   **Yield:** 2 (¾-cup) servings

Raspberries and plums aren't a common combination, but together they create a beverage that refreshes and satisfies. The almond milk tones things down, making this smoothie the perfect addition to your post-op diet.

½ cup unsweetened almond milk

½ cup frozen raspberries

1 cup chopped plums

½ cup ice (optional)

1. In a blender, combine the almond milk, raspberries, plums, and ice (if using) and purée on medium speed until smooth, about 30 seconds.

2. Pour into 2 glasses and enjoy.

3. Store any leftover smoothie in a sealed container, such as a mason jar with a lid, in the refrigerator for up to 2 days. The liquid and solid ingredients will separate and impact the taste and texture, so reblend the smoothie for 10 to 15 seconds before serving.

Post-op tip: If you cannot tolerate fruit skin pieces, peel the plum before chopping and adding to the blender.

Per Serving: Calories: 65; Fat: 1.1g; Protein: 0.9g; Carbs: 14.15g; Fiber: 3.6g; Sugar: 9.9g; Sodium: 48mg

BANANA APPLE FLAX SMOOTHIE

Prep time: 5 minutes   **Yield:** 2 (½-cup) servings

Try this fiber-rich smoothie full of mellow fruity flavor and a pinch of cinnamon. Adding ground flaxseed provides a thick mouthfeel reminiscent of breakfast cereal plus a healthy serving of easily digestible fiber along with omega-3 fatty acids that are beneficial for heart health. This one tastes great warm. After blending, microwave for about a minute and eat with a spoon.

½ cup unsweetened almond milk

½ cup sliced banana

½ cup peeled and chopped apple

1 tablespoon ground flaxseed

¼ teaspoon ground cinnamon plus more, as desired

1. In a blender, combine the almond milk, banana, apple, flaxseed, and cinnamon and purée on low speed until smooth, about 30 seconds.

2. Pour into 2 glasses and enjoy.

3. Store any leftover smoothie in a sealed container, such as a mason jar with a lid, in the refrigerator for up to 2 days. The liquid and solid ingredients will separate and impact the taste and texture, so reblend the smoothie for 10 to 15 seconds before serving.

Post-op tip: If you are having trouble tolerating large amounts of fiber in one sitting, go ahead and omit the flaxseed from the recipe. It will still taste great.

Per Serving: Calories: 76; Fat: 2.26g; Protein: 1.4g; Carbs: 14g; Fiber: 2.6g; Sugar: 6.6g; Sodium: 48mg

CITRUS BANANA SMOOTHIE

Prep time: 5 minutes   **Yield:** 2 (½-cup) servings

Sometimes sticking with the classics can be just what the doctor ordered. Orange and banana are a match made in heaven, and if you like, you can add some plain nonfat Greek yogurt or more banana to make it creamier and even thicker. Keep in mind, though, that those will also add more carbohydrates to the final smoothie.

½ cup unsweetened almond milk

¼ teaspoon orange zest

¼ cup freshly squeezed orange juice

½ cup sliced banana

1. In a blender, combine the almond milk, orange zest, orange juice, and banana and purée on low speed until smooth, 15 to 30 seconds.

2. Pour into 2 glasses and enjoy.

3. Store any leftover smoothie in a sealed container, such as a mason jar with a lid, in the refrigerator for up to 2 days. The liquid and solid ingredients will separate and impact the taste and texture, so reblend the smoothie for 10 to 15 seconds before serving.

Prep tip: To make it easier to squeeze the juice from an orange, use a handheld citrus squeezer (or a juicer if you have one). Try to avoid using prepackaged orange juice unless you are sure it contains no added sugar.

Variation tip: Any type of citrus fruit juice and its zest will work in this recipe, such as lemon, lime, or grapefruit.

Per Serving: Calories: 58; Fat: 0.8g; Protein: 0.87g; Carbs: 12.9g; Fiber: 1.2g; Sugar: 7.7g; Sodium: 52mg

BLACKBERRY PEACH SMOOTHIE

Prep time: 3 minutes   **Yield:** 2 (¾-cup) servings

Almond milk is the ingredient that pulls together the flavors of blackberries and peaches. The combination creates a tummy-calming smoothie that works for your post-op needs and tastes like your favorite pie.

1 cup unsweetened almond milk

1 cup frozen sliced peaches

½ cup frozen blackberries

½ teaspoon alcohol-free vanilla extract (optional)

1. In a blender, combine the almond milk, peaches, blackberries, and vanilla (if using) and purée on medium speed until smooth, about 90 seconds.

2. Pour into 2 glasses and enjoy.

3. Store any leftover smoothie in a sealed container, such as a mason jar with a lid, in the refrigerator for up to 2 days. The liquid and solid ingredients will separate and impact the taste and texture, so reblend the smoothie for 10 to 15 seconds before serving.

Prep tip: Feel free to omit the blackberries and add any other berry you have on hand, but keep in mind that this will impact the final flavor of the smoothie.

Variation tip: For a sweeter taste, add 1 teaspoon of your favorite low-calorie sweetener.

Per Serving: Calories: 63.3; Fat: 1g; Protein: 1.1g; Carbs: 13.33g; Fiber: 1.0g; Sugar:10.6 g; Sodium: 63mg

STRAWBERRY PINEAPPLE SMOOTHIE

Prep time: 3 minutes   **Yield:** 2 (¾-cup) servings

For a stomach-calming beverage with a bit of protein to help you hit your daily nutrient needs, try this tropical twist on the average berry smoothie. The natural sweetness of the pineapple is sure to satisfy anyone with a sweet tooth.

½ **cup plain nonfat Greek yogurt**

½ **cup water**

1 cup frozen diced pineapple

½ **cup frozen strawberries**

1. In a blender, combine the yogurt, water, pineapple, and strawberries and purée on medium speed until smooth, about 60 seconds.

2. Pour into 2 glasses and enjoy.

3. Store any leftover smoothie in a sealed container, such as a mason jar with a lid, in the refrigerator for up to 2 days. The liquid and solid ingredients will separate and impact the taste and texture, so reblend the smoothie for 10 to 15 seconds before serving.

Post-op tip: Add more Greek yogurt or mix 1 to 2 tablespoons of protein powder with a little almond milk before blending for extra protein content. Add more water or unsweetened almond milk until the smoothie is pourable. Keep in mind that adding more almond milk will increase the calories of the final smoothie.

Per Serving: Calories: 88; Fat: 0.35g; Protein: 6.9g; Carbs: 15.4g; Fiber: 1.8g; Sugar: 7.4g; Sodium: 24mg

BERRY SPINACH SMOOTHIE

Prep time: 5 minutes   **Yield:** 2 (¾-cup) servings

An easy way to work some greens into your diet, this light and fruity blended beverage will make you forget you're drinking vegetables. Spinach and strawberries provide a powerful mix of antioxidants and fiber to make this a delicious and nutritious smoothie that will help speed your recovery.

½ **cup soy milk**
½ **cup plain nonfat Greek yogurt**
1 **cup frozen strawberries**
1 **cup fresh baby spinach leaves**
1 **teaspoon lemon juice**

1. In a blender, combine the soy milk, yogurt, strawberries, spinach, and lemon juice and purée on medium speed until smooth, about 60 seconds.

2. Pour into 2 glasses and enjoy.

3. Store any leftover smoothie in a sealed container, such as a mason jar with a lid, in the refrigerator for up to 2 days. The liquid and solid ingredients will separate and impact the taste and texture, so reblend the smoothie for 10 to 15 seconds before serving.

Post-op tip: If you have trouble tolerating seeds and veggie pieces, strain the smoothie in a fine-mesh strainer. Keep in mind that this will reduce the yield of this recipe. To increase the protein content, add more yogurt or mix 1 to 2 tablespoons of protein powder with the soy milk before blending.

Per Serving: Calories: 95; Fat: 1.2g; Protein: 8.3g; Carbs: 13.2g; Fiber: 1.7g; Sugar: 7.7g; Sodium: 69mg

ULTIMATE BERRY BLEND SMOOTHIE

Prep time: 5 minutes   **Yield:** 4 (½-cup) servings

A quartet of everyone's favorite berries combines with the mellow flavor of coconut yogurt to create a smoothie with just the right amount of sweetness. This smoothie is thick and fiber- and antioxidant-rich to help you through the healing process.

½ cup water

¾ cup unsweetened coconut yogurt

½ cup frozen strawberries

½ cup frozen raspberries

½ cup frozen blueberries

½ cup frozen blackberries

2 teaspoons honey

1. In a blender, combine the water, yogurt, strawberries, raspberries, blueberries, blackberries, and honey and purée on high speed until smooth, about 60 seconds.

2. Pour into glasses and enjoy.

3. Store any leftover smoothie in a sealed container, such as a mason jar with a lid, in the refrigerator for up to 2 days. The liquid and solid ingredients will separate and impact the taste and texture, so reblend the smoothie for 10 to 15 seconds before serving.

Variation tip: For a higher protein content, omit the coconut yogurt and add Greek yogurt instead, though the smoothie will taste more tart.

Per Serving: Calories: 36; Fat: 1.8g; Protein: 0.8g; Carbs: 14.3g; Fiber: 3.6g; Sugar: 8.4g; Sodium: 10mg

GREEN KIWI SPINACH SMOOTHIE

Prep time: 5 minutes   **Yield:** 2 (¾-cup) servings

The slight tart flavor of kiwi helps balance out the bitterness of the spinach, resulting in a smoothie that is vitamin C-rich and very delicious. This is a good choice when you want a lot of hydration while getting in a dose of antioxidants to help soothe your gut and heal your body.

½ **cup water**

1 **cup frozen chopped spinach**

1 **cup peeled and chopped kiwi**

1. In a blender, combine the water, spinach, and kiwi and purée on low speed until smooth, 15 to 30 seconds.

2. Pour into 2 glasses and enjoy.

3. Store any leftover smoothie in a sealed container, such as a mason jar with a lid, in the refrigerator for up to 2 days. The liquid and solid ingredients will separate and impact the taste and texture, so reblend the smoothie for 10 to 15 seconds before serving.

Post-op tip: If you cannot yet tolerate seeds or raw vegetable pieces, you may want to strain this smoothie through a fine-mesh strainer. The yield will likely be cut in half, and the fiber content will be greatly reduced.

Variation tip: Add some Greek yogurt to boost the protein and create a thicker consistency, though it will increase the calories of the smoothie. If you choose to strain out the seeds and spinach pieces, strain the mixture first, discard the solids, and pour the liquid into the blender with the yogurt.

Per Serving: Calories: 75; Fat: .84g; Protein: 3.8g; Carbs: 15.9g; Fiber: 5g; Sugar: 8.6g; Sodium: 62mg

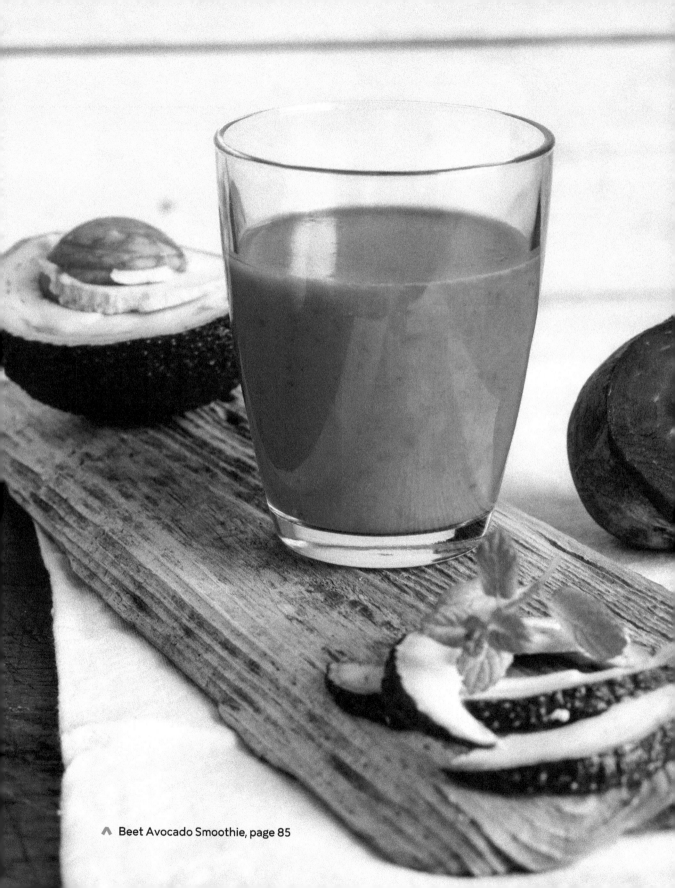

Beet Avocado Smoothie, page 85

5
SAVORY

Smoothies don't have to be sweet! Change up your smoothie routine with some savory flavors. These smoothie recipes contain a lot of veggies with a bit of fruit, herbs, and warming spices and are blended into a smooth, easy-to-sip form. Adjust the amounts of herbs, spices, and salt to your preference because your taste buds may have changed a bit after surgery. And if you're dairy free, you can replace any yogurt in the recipes with a mixture of a bit of protein powder and plant-based milk to maintain a similar nutrient profile.

TOMATO BASIL SMOOTHIE

Prep time: 5 minutes **Yield:** 2 (½-cup) servings

Bring the flavor of *Italia* into your smoothie routine with this refreshing herbal blend. The addition of Greek yogurt brings a rich protein content and a smooth consistency. If you are avoiding dairy, add the same quantity of silken tofu to maintain the protein content. Greek yogurt and silken tofu each contain 15 to 20 grams of protein per cup.

½ cup plain nonfat Greek yogurt

1 cup chopped Roma tomatoes

1 teaspoon chopped fresh basil

¼ teaspoon salt plus more, as desired

Pinch freshly ground black pepper (optional)

1. In a blender, combine the yogurt, tomatoes, basil, salt, and pepper (if using) and purée on low speed until smooth, about 30 seconds.

2. Pour into 2 glasses and enjoy.

3. Store any leftover smoothie in a sealed container, such as a mason jar with a lid, in the refrigerator for up to 2 days. The liquid and solid ingredients will separate and impact the taste and texture, so reblend the smoothie for 10 to 15 seconds before serving.

Prep tip: If fresh tomatoes aren't accessible or you just prefer to have a shelf-stable option on hand, feel free to use canned low-sodium diced tomatoes in this recipe.

Per Serving: Calories: 55; Fat: .43g; Protein: 7.2g; Carbs: 6g; Fiber: 1.3g; Sugar: 4.4g; Sodium: 318mg

GARLIC GREEN
GARDEN SMOOTHIE

Prep time: 5 minutes   **Yield:** 2 (1-cup) servings

This isn't your typical green smoothie. It combines four green veggies with the potent flavors of garlic and a touch of dill that will give you a unique beverage that can be enjoyed cold or warm and is sure to satisfy any cravings you might have for "real" food. Replace the yogurt with silken tofu to maintain a similar texture and protein level without the dairy.

½ cup plain nonfat
Greek yogurt

½ cup unsweetened
almond milk

1 cup fresh baby
spinach leaves

1 cup peeled, seeded,
and chopped
cucumber

½ cup seeded and
chopped green
bell pepper

¼ cup peeled, seeded,
and mashed avocado

2 teaspoons
garlic powder

1 teaspoon chopped
fresh dill

¼ teaspoon salt plus
more, as desired

1. In a blender, combine the yogurt, almond milk, spinach, cucumber, bell pepper, avocado, garlic powder, dill, and salt and purée on medium speed until smooth, about 60 seconds.

2. Pour into 2 glasses and enjoy.

3. Store any leftover smoothie in a sealed container, such as a mason jar with a lid, in the refrigerator for up to 2 days. The liquid and solid ingredients will separate and impact the taste and texture, so reblend the smoothie for 10 to 15 seconds before serving.

Post-op tip: If you are having a hard time tolerating fiber-rich foods after surgery, divide the smoothie into smaller serving sizes.

Per Serving: Calories: 126; Fat: 4.8g; Protein: 9.1g; Carbs: 12.7g; Fiber: 3.3g; Sugar: 4.2g; Sodium: 385mg

BLOODY MARY SMOOTHIE

Prep time: 5 minutes   **Yield:** 2 (½-cup) servings

Drink up this morning cocktail smoothie that is reminiscent of the classic Bloody Mary minus the stomach-irritating spirits. The possible variations here are nearly limitless, so try adding more citrus juice or substituting other seasonings depending on the flavors you like. You can also add ice to the blender if a colder drink is more to your liking.

1 cup chopped Roma tomatoes

½ teaspoon chopped fresh basil

6 pitted green olives

1 teaspoon lemon juice

½ teaspoon garlic powder

¼ teaspoon salt plus more, as desired

Pinch freshly ground black pepper

1. In a blender, combine the tomatoes, basil, olives, lemon juice, garlic powder, salt, and pepper and purée on low speed until smooth, about 45 seconds.

2. Pour into 2 glasses and enjoy.

3. Store any leftover smoothie in a sealed container, such as a mason jar with a lid, in the refrigerator for up to 2 days. The liquid and solid ingredients will separate and impact the taste and texture, so reblend the smoothie for 10 to 15 seconds before serving.

Post-op tip: If you want to boost the protein, mix 1 to 2 tablespoons of unflavored protein powder with a creamy liquid like unsweetened soy milk or almond milk before blending. Please note that adding any soy or almond milk will increase the calories a bit.

Per Serving: Calories: 32; Fat: 1.4g; Protein: 1.1g; Carbs: 4.7g; Fiber: 1.5g; Sugar: 2.5g; Sodium: 423mg

TOMATO PARMESAN SMOOTHIE

Prep time: 5 minutes   **Yield:** 2 (½-cup) servings

This unique smoothie is for anyone who loves pizza but wants to avoid bread or can't tolerate the texture during the post-op recovery. Believe it or not, this smoothie can fill the void. The best part is that the cottage cheese gives it a rich protein content, so it makes a great meal replacement.

½ cup **4 percent milkfat cottage cheese**
1 cup **chopped Roma tomatoes**
1 tablespoon **grated parmesan cheese**
½ **cup ice**

1. In a blender, combine the cottage cheese, tomatoes, parmesan cheese, and ice and purée on medium speed until smooth, 30 to 60 seconds.

2. Pour into 2 glasses and enjoy.

3. Store any leftover smoothie in a sealed container, such as a mason jar with a lid, in the refrigerator for up to 2 days. The liquid and solid ingredients will separate and impact the taste and texture, so reblend the smoothie for 10 to 15 seconds before serving.

Post-op tip: If you can't tolerate much fat, use a lower-fat cottage cheese product or replace the cottage cheese with silken tofu.

Per Serving: Calories: 78; Fat: 2.7g; Protein: 7g; Carbs: 5.6g; Fiber: 1.1g; Sugar: 3.8g; Sodium: 215mg

SAVORY CHILI CUCUMBER SMOOTHIE

Prep time: 5 minutes   **Yield:** 2 (½-cup) servings

Reminiscent of cooling cucumber dips like tzatziki or raita, this smoothie offers the refreshing mild flavor of cucumber with the addition of just a bit of heat. If cayenne pepper is too intense for your taste, try using paprika. And if you are craving more heat, go ahead and add your favorite hot sauce. The yogurt cools everything off so it won't irritate your healing gut while contributing some filling protein.

¼ **cup plain nonfat Greek yogurt**

1 **cup peeled, seeded, and chopped cucumber**

½ **teaspoon cayenne pepper**

⅛ **teaspoon salt**

½ **cup ice**

1. In a blender, combine the yogurt, cucumber, cayenne, salt, and ice and purée on medium speed until smooth, about 60 seconds.

2. Pour into 2 glasses and enjoy.

3. Store any leftover smoothie in a sealed container, such as a mason jar with a lid, in the refrigerator for up to 2 days. The liquid and solid ingredients will separate and impact the taste and texture, so reblend the smoothie for 10 to 15 seconds before serving.

Post-op tip: If you want to boost the protein content of this shake, add more Greek yogurt or some silken tofu. Note that adding any ingredients will increase the yield of the recipe, possibly alter the texture or thickness of the smoothie, and increase the calories. Also, consuming spicy foods may not be preferable in the early stages after surgery, so don't add more spices to this smoothie for at least 3 months post-op or as recommended by your surgeon.

Per Serving: Calories: 27; Fat: 1.7g; Protein: 3.6g; Carbs: 2.8g; Fiber: .59g; Sugar: 2.4g; Sodium: 158mg

GAZPACHO-STYLE SMOOTHIE

Prep time: 5 minutes   **Yield:** 2 (1-cup) servings

This blend provides the refreshing veggie flavors of gazpacho, but with the addition of yogurt to provide extra protein and a creamier consistency, which will be better for the post-op stomach. One sip of this savory smoothie will remind you of a breezy, warm summer afternoon when vegetables are at their peak.

½ cup plain nonfat
   Greek yogurt
½ cup chopped
   Roma tomatoes
½ cup peeled, seeded,
   and chopped
   cucumber
½ cup seeded and
   chopped bell pepper
¼ cup chopped
   yellow onion
¼ teaspoon salt
Pinch freshly ground
   black pepper
1 cup ice

1. In a blender, combine the yogurt, tomatoes, cucumber, bell pepper, onion, salt, black pepper, and ice and purée on medium speed until smooth, about 60 seconds.

2. Pour into 2 glasses and enjoy.

3. Store any leftover smoothie in a sealed container, such as a mason jar with a lid, in the refrigerator for up to 2 days. The liquid and solid ingredients will separate and impact the taste and texture, so reblend the smoothie for 10 to 15 seconds before serving.

Prep tip: If you prefer a smoother texture, add a few tablespoons of mashed avocado and blend for an additional 30 seconds. Two tablespoons of avocado will add about 50 calories, 1 net gram of carbohydrate, and 4 grams of fat.

Per Serving: Calories: 74; Fat: .37g; Protein: 7.6g; Carbs: 8.7g; Fiber: 1.6g; Sugar: 5.9g; Sodium: 318mg

AVOCADO TOMATO SMOOTHIE

Prep time: 5 minutes   **Yield:** 2 (½-cup) servings

Bright tomato flavor pairs wonderfully with the rich consistency of avocado in this refreshing, fiber-rich beverage that is perfect for your post-op diet. Try adding a little chopped fresh basil, oregano, garlic, or cilantro for more complex flavor, if you like.

½ cup plain nonfat
   Greek yogurt
½ cup chopped fresh
   Roma tomatoes
¼ cup peeled, pitted,
   and mashed avocado
⅛ teaspoon salt
½ cup ice

1. In a blender, combine the yogurt, tomatoes, avocado, salt, and ice and purée on low speed until smooth, about 60 seconds.

2. Pour into 2 glasses and enjoy.

3. Store any leftover smoothie in a sealed container, such as a mason jar with a lid, in the refrigerator for up to 2 days. The liquid and solid ingredients will separate and impact the taste and texture, so reblend the smoothie for 10 to 15 seconds before serving.

Prep tip: If you want to save time or prevent any waste from using only part of an avocado, look for packaged mashed avocado in the produce section at some supermarkets, which will keep well in the refrigerator, unopened, for a month or two.

Per Serving: Calories: 91; Fat: 4.5g; Protein: 7.3g; Carbs: 6.4g; Fiber: 2.4g; Sugar: 3.4g; Sodium: 172mg

GREEN DREAM SMOOTHIE

Prep time: 5 minutes   **Yield:** 2 (¾-cup) servings

Whether you enjoy leafy greens or not, you can love them in this delicious and refreshing smoothie that will help you reap the benefits of consuming such nutrient-dense veggies. Cucumber provides a subtly sweet taste, while avocado provides a smooth consistency and filling healthy fat and fiber source that will leave you feeling full and satisfied.

½ cup plain nonfat Greek yogurt

½ cup peeled, pitted, and mashed avocado

½ cup peeled, seeded, and chopped cucumber

2 cups fresh baby spinach leaves

¼ teaspoon salt plus more, as desired

1 cup ice

1. In a blender, combine the yogurt, avocado, cucumber, spinach, salt, and ice and purée on medium speed until smooth, about 60 seconds.

2. Pour into 2 glasses and enjoy.

3. Store any leftover smoothie in a sealed container, such as a mason jar with a lid, in the refrigerator for up to 2 days. The liquid and solid ingredients will separate and impact the taste and texture, so reblend the smoothie for 10 to 15 seconds before serving.

Post-op tip: If you cannot tolerate the raw spinach pieces in your smoothie, use 1 cup of cooked spinach instead of 2 cups raw. For convenience, using cooked frozen spinach is acceptable, or you can blanch or steam raw spinach before blending. Steamed spinach can be stored in a sealed container in the refrigerator for up to 5 days.

Per Serving: Calories: 143; Fat: 8.7g; Protein: 8.6g; Carbs: 9.8g; Fiber: 4.5g; Sugar: 2.8g; Sodium: 351mg

GARDEN VEGGIE SALAD SMOOTHIE

Prep time: 5 minutes   **Yield:** 2 (1-cup) servings

Here's another way to get your vegetables if you can't yet tolerate the texture of raw veggies. Greek yogurt and dill form the creamy (and tasty) "dressing" that's blended with tomato, bell pepper, spinach, and carrot "salad." You'll get all the protein and vitamins you need in one refreshing beverage that is kind to your tummy. I call for frozen carrots because they are usually blanched, and when blended, they will have a less gritty texture than if you tried to blend raw carrots.

½ cup plain nonfat Greek yogurt

½ cup chopped Roma tomatoes

½ cup seeded and chopped bell pepper

2 cups fresh baby spinach leaves

¼ cup chopped yellow onion

½ cup chopped frozen carrots

½ teaspoon chopped dill

¼ teaspoon salt

1 cup ice

1. In a blender, combine the yogurt, tomatoes, bell pepper, spinach, onion, carrots, salt, and ice and purée on medium speed until smooth, about 60 seconds.

2. Pour into 2 glasses and enjoy.

3. Store any leftover smoothie in a sealed container, such as a mason jar with a lid, in the refrigerator for up to 2 days. The liquid and solid ingredients will separate and impact the taste and texture, so reblend the smoothie for 10 to 15 seconds before serving.

Prep tip: To produce an even smoother consistency, you can steam or boil the carrots until tender, 4 to 5 minutes, before blending. You can store steamed carrots in the refrigerator in a sealed container for up to 5 days.

Per Serving: Calories: 86; Fat: .31g; Protein: 8.7g; Carbs: 12.6g; Fiber: 3g; Sugar: 6g; Sodium: 372mg

CARROT CAKE SMOOTHIE

Prep time: 5 minutes   **Yield:** 2 (¾-cup) servings

If you want your cake but can't eat it because of sugar intolerance, you'll love this low-carb, drinkable version of carrot cake. Feel free to add a bit of cream cheese in addition to the yogurt to get a reminder of the typical frosting choice in this classic cake.

1 cup chopped
  frozen carrots
½ cup plain nonfat
  Greek yogurt
½ cup peeled and
  chopped apple
½ cup unsweetened
  almond milk
2 teaspoons
  alcohol-free
  vanilla extract
1 teaspoon ground
  cinnamon

1. In a blender, combine the carrots, yogurt, apple, almond milk, vanilla, and cinnamon and purée on high speed until smooth, about 60 seconds.

2. Pour into 2 glasses and enjoy.

3. Store any leftover smoothie in a sealed container, such as a mason jar with a lid, in the refrigerator for up to 2 days. The liquid and solid ingredients will separate and impact the taste and texture, so reblend the smoothie for 10 to 15 seconds before serving.

Post-op tip: For more protein, replace the almond milk with soy milk. It won't affect the flavor profile much.

Prep tip: To make a sweeter-tasting smoothie, use sweetened almond milk, which typically adds about 6 grams of sugar per cup.

Per Serving: Calories: 101; Fat: 1.2g; Protein: 7.2g; Carbs: 12.3g; Fiber: 1.7g; Sugar: 9g; Sodium: 115mg

CARROT ORANGE GINGER SMOOTHIE

Prep time: 5 minutes   **Yield:** 2 (¾-cup) servings

Ginger is great for soothing a variety of gastrointestinal discomforts and is also a delicious accompaniment to carrots. Refreshing and slightly spicy, this smoothie is brightly flavored and great for your post-op gut. If you use fresh carrots instead of frozen, be sure to steam or blanch them until tender before blending to create the smoothest consistency.

½ cup soy milk

½ cup plain nonfat
  Greek yogurt

¼ teaspoon orange zest

¼ cup freshly squeezed
  orange juice

1 cup chopped
  frozen carrots

¼ teaspoon
  ground ginger

1. In a blender, combine the soy milk, yogurt, orange zest, orange juice, carrots, and ginger and purée on high speed until smooth, about 60 seconds.

2. Pour into 2 glasses and enjoy.

3. Store any leftover smoothie in a sealed container, such as a mason jar with a lid, in the refrigerator for up to 2 days. The liquid and solid ingredients will separate and impact the taste and texture, so reblend the smoothie for 10 to 15 seconds before serving.

Prep tip: Try using ½ teaspoon of minced fresh ginger instead of the ground ginger for a zingier ginger taste.

Per Serving: Calories: 105; Fat: 1.2g; Protein: 8.8g; Carbs: 10.5g; Fiber: <1g; Sugar: 9.8g; Sodium: 97mg

BEET AVOCADO SMOOTHIE

Prep time: 5 minutes   **Yield:** 2 (¾-cup) servings

If you've ever heard the instruction "eat the rainbow," you may know that different-colored foods provide different nutritional benefits. This beautiful pink-hued smoothie has a subtly sweet and fresh taste with a smooth texture that will help cleanse your palate and satisfy your appetite at meal or snack time while being easy on your post-surgery gut. The beets also provide a rich antioxidant component that can improve vascular health, while the avocado offers healthy fat and a silky-smooth texture. Try adding a few fresh mint leaves for a special treat.

½ cup soy milk

½ cup peeled, pitted, and mashed avocado

1 cup peeled and chopped raw beets

½ cup peeled and chopped apple

1. In a blender, combine the soy milk, avocado, beets, and apple and purée on high speed until smooth, about 60 seconds.

2. Pour into 2 glasses and enjoy.

3. Store any leftover smoothie in a sealed container, such as a mason jar with a lid, in the refrigerator for up to 2 days. The liquid and solid ingredients will separate and impact the taste and texture, so reblend the smoothie for 10 to 15 seconds before serving.

Post-op tip: Increase the protein by adding 1 to 2 tablespoons of unflavored protein powder or some silken tofu.

Prep tip: Blanch the beets or cook them until tender, 4 to 5 minutes, for a smoother consistency.

Per Serving: Calories: 167; Fat: 10.5g; Protein: 3g; Carbs: 18g; Fiber: 6.2g; Sugar: 10g; Sodium: 86mg g

TURMERIC TOFU SMOOTHIE

Prep time: 3 minutes   **Yield:** 2 (¾-cup) servings

Tofu may not seem like an obvious choice for a smoothie, but one taste of this anti-inflammatory refreshment will change your mind. The silken type of tofu brings a super-smooth consistency and a protein punch, while antioxidant-rich turmeric lends a pleasantly bitter note. Soy milk and vanilla add a subtle sweetness that makes this mild smoothie go down easy for those healing from surgery.

½ **cup soy milk**

1 **cup silken tofu**

1 **teaspoon alcohol-free vanilla extract**

¼ **teaspoon ground turmeric**

1. In a blender, combine the soy milk, tofu, vanilla, and turmeric and purée on low speed until smooth, about 30 seconds.

2. Pour into 2 glasses and enjoy.

3. Store any leftover smoothie in a sealed container, such as a mason jar with a lid, in the refrigerator for up to 2 days. The liquid and solid ingredients will separate and impact the taste and texture, so reblend the smoothie for 10 to 15 seconds before serving.

Prep tip: Add more alcohol-free vanilla extract to make this smoothie slightly sweeter, if you like.

Per Serving: Calories: 123; Fat: 4.9g; Protein: 13.6g; Carbs: 7.5g; Fiber: .2g; Sugar: 2.5g; Sodium: 29mg

SPICED TOFU SMOOTHIE

Prep time: 5 minutes   **Yield:** 2 (½-cup) servings

The warming spices of paprika and cinnamon in this smoothie offer flavor without upsetting your post-op stomach. The bell pepper provides a fresh flavor along with some color, and the soy milk gives the recipe a needed protein boost.

1 cup silken tofu
¼ cup soy milk
¼ cup seeded and chopped green bell pepper
¼ teaspoon paprika
¼ teaspoon ground cinnamon

1. In a blender, combine the tofu, soy milk, bell pepper, paprika, and cinnamon and purée on low speed until smooth, about 30 seconds.

2. Pour into 2 glasses and enjoy.

3. Store any leftover smoothie in a sealed container, such as a mason jar with a lid, in the refrigerator for up to 2 days. The liquid and solid ingredients will separate and impact the taste and texture, so reblend the smoothie for 10 to 15 seconds before serving.

Prep tip: Feel free to add chopped sweet pepper instead of green bell pepper if you prefer a sweeter flavor profile.

Per Serving: Calories: 110; Fat: 4.5g; Protein: 13g; Carbs: 7g; Fiber: .83g; Sugar: 1.4g; Sodium: 15mg

BUTTERNUT SQUASH CURRY SMOOTHIE

Prep time: 5 minutes   **Yield:** 2 (1-cup) servings

Discover the flavors of fall in this delicious savory and satisfying smoothie with a touch of spice. Butternut squash provides a smooth and fiber-rich foundation, and the addition of Greek yogurt enhances this smoothie with a creamy, protein-rich finish that balances out the bold taste of the bell pepper and curry powder. This smoothie is delicious warmed or chilled.

½ cup plain nonfat
    Greek yogurt
1 cup canned or frozen
    unsweetened butter-
    nut squash purée
½ cup peeled and
    chopped apples
¼ cup seeded and
    chopped bell pepper
½ teaspoon ground
    cinnamon
¼ teaspoon
    curry powder

1. In a blender, combine the yogurt, butternut squash, apple, bell pepper, cinnamon, and curry powder and purée on medium speed until smooth, 30 to 60 seconds.

2. Pour into 2 glasses and enjoy.

3. Store any leftover smoothie in a sealed container, such as a mason jar with a lid, in the refrigerator for up to 2 days. The liquid and solid ingredients will separate and impact the taste and texture, so reblend the smoothie for 10 to 15 seconds before serving.

Prep tip: To warm the smoothie, pour it into a small saucepan and heat over low heat for 3 to 5 minutes, or pour it into a microwave-safe bowl and microwave for 1 minute or until hot.

Variation tip: For a more filling beverage, add some cottage cheese or extra yogurt. This will add extra protein, but be aware that this will also add carbohydrates and calories.

Per Serving: Calories: 108; Fat: 0.62g; Protein: 7.7g; Carbs: 19.5g; Fiber: 2.8g; Sugar: 9g; Sodium: 28mg

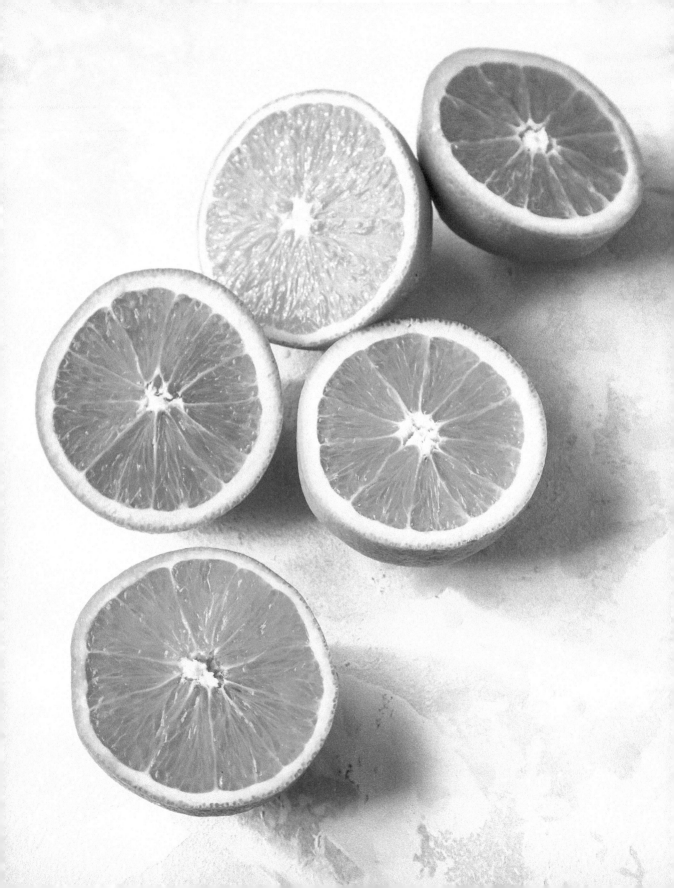

Measurement Conversions

	U.S. Standard	U.S. Standard (ounces)	Metric (approximate)
LIQUID	2 tablespoons	1 fl. oz.	30 mL
	¼ cup	2 fl. oz.	60 mL
	½ cup	4 fl. oz.	120 mL
	1 cup	8 fl. oz.	240 mL
	1½ cups	12 fl. oz.	355 mL
	2 cups or 1 pint	16 fl. oz.	475 mL
	4 cups or 1 quart	32 fl. oz.	1 L
	1 gallon	128 fl. oz.	4 L
DRY	⅛ teaspoon	—	0.5 mL
	¼ teaspoon	—	1 mL
	½ teaspoon	—	2 mL
	¾ teaspoon	—	4 mL
	1 teaspoon	—	5 mL
	1 tablespoon	—	15 mL
	¼ cup	—	59 mL
	⅓ cup	—	79 mL
	½ cup	—	118 mL
	⅔ cup	—	156 mL
	¾ cup	—	177 mL
	1 cup	—	235 mL
	2 cups or 1 pint	—	475 mL
	3 cups	—	700 mL
	4 cups or 1 quart	—	1 L
	½ gallon	—	2 L
	1 gallon	—	4 L

OVEN TEMPERATURES

Fahrenheit	Celsius (approximate)
250°F	120°C
300°F	150°C
325°F	165°C
350°F	180°C
375°F	190°C
400°F	200°C
425°F	220°C
450°F	230°C

WEIGHT EQUIVALENTS

U.S. Standard	Metric (approximate)
½ ounce	15 g
1 ounce	30 g
2 ounces	60 g
4 ounces	115 g
8 ounces	225 g
12 ounces	340 g
16 ounces or 1 pound	455 g

References

Ajami, Marjan, et al. "Effects of Stevia on Glycemic and Lipid Profile of Type 2 Diabetic Patients: A Randomized Controlled Trial." *Avicenna Journal of Phytomedicine* 10, no. 2 (March–April 2020): 118–27.

American Society for Metabolic and Bariatric Surgery. "Care Pathway Development for Laparoscopic Sleeve Gastrectomy." Accessed November 2021. ASMBS.org/app/uploads/2016/09/Telem-et-al_LSG-Pathway_2016_Final.pdf.

American Society for Metabolic and Bariatric Surgery. "FAQs of Bariatric Surgery." Accessed November 2021. ASMBS.org/patients/faqs-of-bariatric-surgery.

American Society for Metabolic and Bariatric Surgery. "Life after Bariatric Surgery." Accessed November 2021. ASMBS.org/patients/life-after-bariatric-surgery.

Bartolotto, Carole. "Does Consuming Sugar and Artificial Sweeteners Change Taste Preferences?" *The Permanente Journal* 19, no. 3 (Summer 2015): 81–84. doi.org/10.7812/TPP/14-229.

Cleveland Clinic Florida Bariatric & Metabolic Institute Department of General and Vascular Surgery. "Nutrition Manual." Accessed November 2021. my.ClevelandClinic.org/-/scassets/files/org/florida/digestive-diseases/bariatric_nutrition_manual.ashx?la=en.

Dagen, Shiri Sherf, et al. "Nutritional Recommendations for Adult Bariatric Surgery Patients: Clinical Practice." *Advances in Nutrition* 8, no. 2 (March 2017): 382–94. doi.org/10.3945/an.116.014258.

Farhat, Grace, Victoria Berset, and Lauren Moore. "Effects of Stevia Extract on Postprandial Glucose Response, Satiety and Energy Intake: A Three-Arm Crossover Trial." *Nutrients* 11, no. 12 (December 12, 2019): 3036. doi.org/10.3390/nu11123036.

Johns Hopkins Medicine. "Nutrition Guidelines for Weight Loss Surgery." Accessed November 2021. HopkinsMedicine.org/bariatrics/_documents/nutrition-guidelines-for-weight-loss-surgery.pdf.

Kanerva, Nora, et al. "Changes in Total Energy Intake and Macronutrient Composition after Bariatric Surgery Predict Long-Term Weight Outcome: Findings from the Swedish Obese Subjects (SOS) Study." *The American Journal of Clinical Nutrition* 106, no. 1 (July 2017): 136–45. doi.org/10.3945/ajcn.116.149112.

Pham, Hung, et al. "The Effects of a Whey Protein and Guar Gum-Containing Preload on Gastric Emptying, Glycaemia, Small Intestinal Absorption and Blood Pressure in Healthy Older Subjects." *Nutrients* 11, no. 11 (November 5, 2019): 2666. doi.org/10.3390/nu11112666.

The Mayo Clinic. "Dumping Syndrome." Accessed November 2019. MayoClinic.org/diseases-conditions/dumping-syndrome/symptoms-causes/syc-20371915.

Tufts Medical Center. "Guide for Eating after Gastric Bypass Surgery." Accessed November 2021. TuftsMedicalCenter.org/-/media/Brochures/TuftsMC/Patient-Care-Services/Departments-and-Services/Weight-and-Wellness-Center/GBP-Diet-Manual12611.ashx?la=en&hash=29F5FC8CE082A84BBD66A46335C50C23B8042A29.

Wen, Huaixiu. "Erythritol Attenuates Postprandial Blood Glucose by Inhibiting α-Glucosidase." *Journal of Agricultural and Food Chemistry* 66, no. 6 (February 14, 2018): 1401–7. doi.org/10.1021/acs.jafc.7b05033.

Index

Acknowledgments

I would like to thank my editor, Anne Goldberg, and the Callisto Media publishing team for their help in the creation of this cookbook. I am very grateful for this experience and really enjoyed developing the recipes for this book.

About the Author

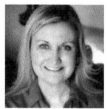 **STACI GULBIN,** MS, MEd, RD, has been a registered dietitian since 2010 and also works as a freelance writer and health editor. Besides blogging on her website, LighttrackNutrition.com, she enjoys the outdoors, cooking, and gardening. She has been a featured expert in online publications like *Shape, Health,* and *Eat This Not That.* Staci holds graduate degrees in Human Nutrition and Nutrition Education from Columbia University's Institute of Human Nutrition and Teacher's College, Columbia University, respectively.

Printed in the USA
CPSIA information can be obtained
at www.ICGtesting.com
CBHW081240200224
4500CB00003B/12